DISABILITY AND SOCIETY: EMERGING ISSUES AND INSIGHTS BAR

LONGMAN SOCIOLOGY SERIES

Disability and Society: Emerging Issues and Insights

edited by Len Barton

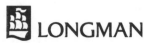

Addison Wesley Longman Limited
Edinburgh Gate
Harlow
Essex
CM20 2JE, England
and Associated Companies throughout the world.

*Published in the United States of America
by Longman Publishing, New York*

First published 1996
Second impression 1998

ISBN 0 582 291666 PPR

British Library Cataloguing-in-Publication Data

A catalogue record for this book is
available from the British Library

Library of Congress Cataloging-in-Publication Data

Disability and society : emerging issues and insights / L. Barton
(ed.)
p.   cm. – (Longman sociology series)
Includes bibliographical references and index.
ISBN 0–582–29166–6
1. Sociology of disability. I. Barton, Len. II. Series.
HV1568.D565 1996
362.4 – dc20   95–46007
                                                                      CIP

Set in 10/11 Times by 5
Printed in Malaysia, TCP

CONTENTS

SERIES EDITOR'S PREFACE

The Longman Sociology Series aims to provide an alternative to the standard texts in the field. Although most of the books in the series are designed with sociology undergraduates in mind, the editors will include books that are of wider interest, both to students, researchers and scholars in cognate fields and to a more general readership who actively use the social sciences.

The series is forward looking and reflects key controversies and debates in sociology and social policy in the 1990s. Each book will be theoretically informed, use new empirical material and have some relevance to political and social policy. The focus of each volume will be upon theoretically informed work. As the volumes are intended for an international audience they frequently contain comparative material.

As the shape, substance, style and content of sociological research changes, it also needs to be reflected in published work so that research findings are accessible to a wide audience and can be disseminated to a new generation of students taking sociological courses.

This volume breaks new ground by examining the debate about disability issues. In particular, the authors suggest ways in which sociologists can contribute to an understanding of disability, help to develop policy and challenge and change current practice. Overall, this collection of essays demonstrates how sociological theory and research can be used to advance our understanding of an important issue for contemporary society and lead to policy development. The essays will lead to a range of further debates and in turn help to firmly establish the study of disability on the discipline's research agenda.

Robert G. Burgess,
University of Warwick

PREFACE

This book represents an attempt to encourage the sociological study of disability. The chapters to this book arose from an invitation only seminar which I organised in October 1994. The intention of the seminar was to reconsider both the existing state of sociological analyses concerned with disability issues as well as attempt to identify possible future directions.

Whilst by no means exhausting the numbers or questioning the influence of sociologists who have been associated with this area of study, nationally and internationally, nevertheless, the overall contribution to such sociological developments by the authors in this volume has been significant.

One of the unique features of the seminar was the drawing together of disabled and non-disabled sociologists. The debates were stimulating, lively and refreshingly open. Agreements and disagreements were identified with some of the latter remaining unresolved. Overall the time together was an important learning experience, strengthening our understandings, making us aware of our limitations as sociologists as well as providing an opportunity for us to learn to respect one another.

The chapters in this volume are offered with the hope that they will in some small way inspire, challenge and encourage other students, researchers and academics to both see the importance of the question of disability and respond to some of the issues, insights and questions which these chapters provide.

Len Barton,
June 1995

ACKNOWLEDGEMENTS

This volume is a testimony to the vital importance of debate in the struggle for ideas and insights relating to the issue of disability. It is also a reminder of the necessity of support and friendship of those involved in the difficult struggle for an inclusive society. We need each other and have much to learn from one another.

I would, therefore, like to thank all the contributors for their crucial involvement in the production of this volume. They kept to very tight deadlines and responded so willingly to comments on their chapters.

Thanks also to Bob Burgess who supported the initial idea of such a volume and continued to express keenness and constructive help.

Finally, thanks to the editorial staff at Longman, for their continued support and encouragement.

CONTRIBUTORS

Paul Abberley taught full time at the University of The West of England for 17 years. He now works part-time, teaching a course in Disability Studies in the Department of Sociology at the University of Bristol. He has been writing in this area since 1985, and has published a number of papers and reviews. He is a member of the editorial board of *Disability and Society* and has been a management committee member and sometime chairperson of the Avon Coalition of Disabled People. In 1992–3 he was consultant to a Policy Studies Institute research project on the Independent Living Fund.

Colin Barnes is a disabled writer and activist with a congenital visual impairment. Besides teaching disability studies in the School of Sociology and Social Policy at the University of Leeds, he is Research Director for the School's Disability Research Unit, Honorary Research Director for the British Council of Organisations of Disabled People (BCODP), and an executive editor of the international journal *Disability and Society*.

Len Barton teaches on MEd and MA courses in the Division of Education, University of Sheffield. He is the founder of the International Journal *Disability & Society*. His research interests include a socio-political approach to disability, and inclusive education.

Tim Booth is a Reader in Social Policy in the Department of Sociological Studies at Sheffield University. He has written and researched widely in the learning difficulties field. His most recent publications include *Outward Bound: Relocation and Community Care for People with Learning Difficulties* (Open University Press 1990), and *Parenting Under Pressure: Mothers and Fathers with Learning Difficulties* (Open University Press 1994). He is currently engaged on an action research project, funded by the Joseph Rowntree Foundation, which aims to develop a locally based advocacy support network for parents who have learning difficulties.

Robert F. Drake is a lecturer in social policy at Swansea University and an honorary research fellow in the University of Cardiff. His research interests include the voluntary sector and the social model of disability. He has contributed to journals such as *Critical Social Policy* and *Disability & Society*, and has recently been engaged in work with the Welsh Health Planning Forum.

Gillian Fulcher is an Associate in the Department of Anthropology and Sociology, Monash University, and an independent researcher. She has taught sociology at Monash University, and researched disability issues since 1983 when she was seconded to the Victorian Department of Education as main writer for a Ministerial Review of Educational Services for the Disabled. Her most recent research is with the Royal Melbourne Institute of Technology on communication and severe disability.

Alan Hurst is Professor in the Department of Education Studies at the University of Central Lancashire and is also an Adviser for Disabled Students. Currently he is senior Vice-Chair of Skill: National Bureau for Students with Disabilities and is a member of the HEFC(E) Advisory Group on Widening Participation. His research interests concern disability and higher education and he hopes to publish a collection of papers about policies and provision in other countries soon.

Mike Oliver is Professor of Disability Studies at the University of Greenwich. He has written extensively on all aspects of disability including *The Politics of Disablement* (Macmillan 1990) and *Understanding Disability: From Theory to Practice* (1995). He has been an activist in the disabled people's movement for the past 20 years and served on several major reviews in health and education. He is currently working on a recent history of the disabled people's movement.

Susan Peters is Associate Professor in the Departments of Teacher Education and Special Education at Michigan State University, as well as Core Faculty Member for African Studies Programmes, MSU. Susan's scholarly publications and research interests focus on special education and comparative education. In 1993 she was a Fulbright Scholar undertaking teaching and research in Zimbabwe for six months. Susan has served on numerous Boards and Foundations advancing the rights of people with disabilities. She is the past director of a Center for Independent Living in California, and past chairperson of the Michigan State Independent Living Council.

Sheila Riddell is a professor in the Department of Education, University of Stirling. After completing her present degree studies at Bristol University in 1988, she then worked as a Research Fellow at Edinburgh investigating the impact of post-Warnock legislation. She has worked at Stirling University since 1989 and her research interests are mainly concerned with policy relating to special educational needs and gender.

Tom Shakespeare is a research fellow at the University of Leeds. He focuses his research on questions of identity, cultural, political and sexual. Recently he has worked on the implications of Human Genome research, and on the sexual politics of disability. He is involved in the disability movement as an activist and performer within local disability networks, and also through REGARD, the national organisation of disabled lesbians, gay men and bisexual people. He is the proud father of two disabled children.

Roger Slee taught until recently at the Queensland University of Technology in Brisbane, Australia. He is now Head of Department at Goldsmiths College, University of London. He was the Editor of the *Australian Disability Review* and is the Editor of the *International Journal of Inclusive Education*.

PART ONE

Theoretical Developments

This section of the book is concerned with providing some insights into the complex and contentious issue of how sociological theorising has and can continue to contribute to our understanding of disability.

This concern raises several key issues including the form, the purpose, and the outcomes of such sociological enquiries. Integral to this process will be the crucial question of the relationship between the sociologist and the disabled people involved in the research.

In his chapter Barton seeks to identify some of the essential features of a social theory of disability. By positioning the analysis within a concern over human rights, social justice and equity, he argues that part of the sociological task is to highlight and challenge discrimination. He contends that future sociological work needs to have a stronger historically informed base and engage with the serious issue of the politics of difference.

Oliver provides an overview of the historical relationship between sociology and theorising about disability as well as a commentary on the developing links between the two. He proposes a framework for auditing this relationship. Central to his approach is a view of sociology as a critical and emancipatory enterprise. Finally, he discusses the ways in which further developments may take place.

The chapter by Barnes focuses on the socio-political theories of disability and the origins of the oppression of disabled people in western society. He argues that the principal theoretical perspectives on disability have ignored, undervalued and misinterpreted the role of culture in the oppression of disabled people. A materialist account of history is presented which shows that although social responses to impairment are by no means universal, there has been a consistent cultural bias against disabled people throughout recorded history clustered around the myth of the 'body perfect'. This has clear implications for future sociological analyses of social responses to people with impairments.

Finally, Abberley in his chapter highlights the way in which social theories give participation in production a crucial importance in social integration. From this perspective work is viewed as a need and a source of identity. Such theories imply the progressive abolition of impairment as restrictive on the development of people's full human capacities. The total achievement of this aim is, for Abberley, impossible. He contends that in the development of liberative social theories of disablement, we need to draw upon sociological sources which do not equate full humanity with labour.

CHAPTER 1

Sociology and disability: some emerging issues

LEN BARTON

This chapter will briefly consider the sociological contributions to the study of disability. An emphasis will be given to an emancipatory approach to such enquiries as well as to an identification of some specific issues which future work needs to engage with. The sociological task is viewed as contributing both to understanding and changing the social world.

An emancipatory approach

Sociology is an inherently inquisitive and controversial activity. Sociologists are always asking questions, sharpening the focus of concern and providing critiques of existing forms of social conditions and relations. Part of the sociological task is to make connections between, for example, structural conditions and the lived reality of people in particular social settings. In attempting to identify 'several related forms of sensibility' which are viewed as indispensable to the sociological analysis, Giddens maintains that:

sociological analysis can play an emancipatory role in human society. At the same time, sociological analysis teaches sobriety. For although knowledge may be an important adjunct to power, it is not the same as power. And our knowledge of history is always tentative and incomplete.

(1986:13)

We need to remind ourselves as sociologists of the importance of *humility*. Given the profundity of the social issues we face in society today – and disability is clearly one of them – there is no room for complacency and every reason for identifying the limitations of our work, including its partial and incomplete status.

This should not be viewed as a desire for false modesty or the pursuit of a form of subjectivism equivalent to some personal spiritual experience, but rather, a genuine recognition that as sociologists we are always *learning*. We therefore need relationships with 'critical' friends; debate, dialogue and self-criticism are essential ingredients of a healthy sociological diet. A questioning approach to social reality is thus axiomatic to the sociological imagination. This is based upon a conviction that existing social arrangements are neither natural nor proper and are therefore subject to critique and change.

Sociology is often depicted as Giddens notes, in terms of an emancipatory or liberating activity and, therefore, he contends:

Sociology cannot be a neutral intellectual endeavour, indifferent to the practical consequences of its analysis for those whose conduct forms its object of study.

(1986: Preface, Second Edition)

This particular viewpoint raises some significant questions about the complex processes involved in the development and articulation of what Mills (1970) calls, the 'sociological imagination'. This entails the dynamic interplay of biography, context and the values informing sociological reflection. Sociology from this perspective is fundamentally a social act. It also has a particular poignancy in relation to those subjects of study who are disabled and, therefore, experience, in differing degrees of intensity, marginalisation, oppression and vulnerability. To what extent sociologists use their positions and abilities in support of a struggle for change, is a crucial issue needing to be seriously examined. Finally, it not only raises questions about the form and purposes of our work, in the field of disability studies, it has implications for the relationships between disabled and non-disabled sociologists.

An 'emancipatory' approach to the study of disability entails engaging with several key issues. For example, establishing relationships with disabled people, listening to their voice and, in my case, being white, male and non-disabled, raises the following sorts of questions:

What right have I to undertake this work?
What responsibilities arise from the privileges I have as a result of my social position?
How can I use my knowledge and skills to challenge forms of oppression disabled people experience?
Does my writing and speaking reproduce a system of domination or challenge that system?

These questions form part of a complex and unfinished series of concerns. They are important aspects of a challenging learning experience which is both disturbing and enabling. What does it mean for a sociologist to *listen* to the subjects of study? What are the important issues for establishing and maintaining relationships with disabled people, when part of the sociological task involves critically engaging with participants' perspectives? How does the emancipatory practice deal with the conflict of interests the sociologist finds herself in over participants' ignorance, prejudice and reactionary motivations and behaviour? Part of the sociological imagination involves a healthy scepticism and a desire to get beneath surface features to the deep structures of social relations and experience. What does this mean for the sociologist who seeks to take a supportive stance in relation to disabled people?

The emancipatory project does involve issues of relationships and ethics but fundamentally it is about the degree to which the sociological imagination contributes to the *benefit* of disabled people. We need to ask, 'Is this a necessary activity,' and, 'What does it entail and how is it achieved?'

In discussing the question of the relationship between poverty and education, Connell challenges researchers to seriously reconsider the nature and purposes of their activities. He raises some immensely important questions, including:

What kind of research would be useful to a black teenager facing crack and structural unemployment in a Boston apartment, or under smog in Los Angeles? What research would be useful to a Hamilton youth staring at those shrinking steelworks, or a bunch of kids in Alberta wondering where the oil jobs went?

(Connell 1993:123)

He contends that 'educational research' is largely irrelevant and provides little, if any benefit, in meeting the needs of such groups.

Disabled sociologists have been extremely critical of the disabling and offensive nature of much of social science research (Oliver 1992; Abberley 1992). This requires some fundamental changes to the social relations of research production and for researchers as Morris advocates, to seriously engage with such questions as:

Who do I want this research to influence?
Who do I want to be aware of this research?
Who do I want to relate to this research?

(1992a:201–2)

What about our work as sociologists? The emancipatory role is not only concerned with demonstrating different forms of discrimination and under what conditions they develop, but also doing something about it (Oliver 1992). This entails 'overt political struggle against oppressive structures' (Harvey 1990:20).

For Connell this is not for the faint-hearted and is 'deeply uncomfortable research' (1993:124). It does necessitate as Troyna so vividly illustrates, researchers critically engaging with the 'types and configurations of power relations which suffuse researchers' understandings of what 'empowerment' might look like' (1994:20). It is a salutary reminder that intent is no guarantee of outcome (Acker, Barry & Esseveld 1983).

What is important sociologically in relation to disability is that we recognise the profundity of the struggle which is concerned with the realisation of a barrier-free society. According to Giddens 'emancipatory politics makes primary the imperatives of justice, equality and participation' (1991:212). Choice and autonomy are being sought. Freedom and responsibility are viewed in terms of collective, social life. Thus, it is about enabling relationships with others, about life chances and lifestyle. This has critical implications for both the nature of the sociological task and the relationship of the sociologist to the subjects of study.

Sociology and disability

Mainstream sociology has historically shown little interest in the issue of disability. A range of possible reasons can be identified for this situation. Sociologists have tended to accept the dominant hegemony with regard to viewing disability in medical and psychological terms. Thus the issue is perceived as pre- or non-sociological. A great deal of sociological work has been based on the assumption of individuals as 'rational' actors (Barbalet 1993). Individuals categorised in terms of being 'subnormal' or 'mentally handicapped' were excluded from this work or viewed as examples of exotic behaviour (Quicke 1986). Finally, sociological work concerned with the generation of theories of social reproduction and the pursuit of change has ignored the ways in which disabled people operate as a powerful social movement (Barton & Oliver 1992).

Even where the question of disability has been addressed it has not been without some concern. For example, Jenkins (1991) makes hardly any reference to the existing work produced by disabled sociologists. If he was aware of it, he chose not to use it.

A great deal of the sociological work accomplished so far has been undertaken by the contributors to this book. Few of these work within mainstream sociology departments or publish in recognised sociology outlets. It is a sobering thought to consider the limited extent to which this work has had any important impact on the discipline itself.

Sociological analysis has, in the past decade in particular, contributed to the development of a growing body of knowledge and insights. These include:

- The generation of a social theory of disability
- The social construction of categories and the ways in which they are shaped by economic and political influences
- Professional ideologies and practice in relation to how they support vested interests and define definitions of need
- The construction of policy and, for example, the extent to which they serve other purposes than the interests of those they are alleged to support
- Providing accounts of the lived experience of disabled people in particular social settings
- Contributing to the development of enabling forms of methodology and research practice
- Examining the disability movement in terms of a social movement for change (Barton & Tomlinson 1981; 1984; Tomlinson 1982; Bines 1986; Abberley 1987; Fulcher 1989; Oliver 1990; Barnes 1991; Shakespeare 1993).

These are examples of the sociological contribution to providing alternative ways of defining disability and challenging various forms of institutional discrimination. Yet, there is no room for complacency. Much more work needs to be done.

Encouragement can be drawn from the examples of similar concerns being expressed in relation to other disciplines. For example, in a discussion of the potential impact of Disability Studies on Political Science in the USA, Hahn, a disabled political scientist, maintains that the principal perspectives of political science seldom provide any serious successful challenge to the status quo. He contends that:

To the extent that the dominant paradigm of political science precludes the incorporation of insights from multi-disciplinary studies, from disabled persons themselves, or even experts in disability policy, the analysis of disability policy may suffer from a lack of essential information and understanding. Perhaps more significantly, the discipline of political science could be deprived of a rich source of concepts and principles that may assist in the resolution of important research questions beyond the realm of disability policy.

(1993:743)

In his desire to see the development of a less parochial political science and one which is more able to engage with studying the complexities and subtleties of social change, Hahn raises the issue of 'identity politics' and the ways in which disadvantaged groups, including disabled people, have struggled to 'translate previously devalued personal characteristics into a positive source of identity' (p. 749). He believes that a serious consideration of the disability movement and the politics of physical difference could be crucial for the development of the discipline. Similar concerns need to be engaged with in relation to sociology.

Definition, history and difference

How we relate to disabled people is influenced, for example, by our past experience of such encounters and the way in which we define 'disability'. Our definitions are crucial in that they may be part of and further legitimate disabilist assumptions and discriminatory practices. Disabled people have been the recipients of a range of offensive responses by other people. These include, horror, fear, anxiety, hostility, distrust, pity, over-protection and patronising behaviour.

One of the dominant influences shaping both professional and common-sense definitions has been the medical model. This approach as Hahn notes: 'imposes a presumption of biological or physiological inferiority upon disabled persons' (1986:89). It emphasises individual loss or inabilities thereby contributing to a dependency model of disability. Labels such as 'invalid', 'cripple', 'spastic', 'handicapped' and 'retarded' all imply both a functional loss and a lack of worth. Such labels have tended to legitimate individual medical and negative views of disability, to the neglect of other perspectives, in particular, those of disabled people.

Disability is a social and political category in that it entails practices of regulations and struggles for choice, empowerment and rights (Oliver 1989; Fulcher 1989). This approach provides a very different understanding of disability and entails an alternative set of assumptions, priorities and explanations, as Hahn clearly shows. He maintains that:

disability stems from the failure of a structured social environment to adjust to the needs and aspirations of citizens with disabilities *rather* than from the inability of a disabled individual to adapt to the demands of society.

(1986:128)

Being disabled involves experiencing discrimination, vulnerability and abusive assaults upon your self-identity and esteem.

Disability is thus a form of oppression which entails social restrictions, as Oliver has so powerfully argued:

All disabled people experience disability as social restriction whether these restrictions occur as a consequence of inaccessible built environments, questionable notions of intelligence and social competence, the inability of the general public to use sign language, the lack of reading material in Braille or hostile public attitudes to people with non-visible disabilities.

(1990:xiv, Introduction)

This perspective challenges both professional and public perceptions of disability. It involves more than changes to access and resource issues.

In a discussion of changing definitions of difference in relation to the history of people classified as 'mentally handicapped', Ryan and Thomas contend that these definitions:

have always been conceived by others, never are they the expression of a group of people finding their own identity, their own history.

(1980:13)

Rather than seeking an explanation in terms of an individual's inabilities they place the emphasis on the *power* of significant groups in defining the identity of others. In this instance, the outcome of such interventions by professionals has been one of disempowerment, marginalisation and dependency.

Medical values and interpretations have, historically, contributed to a view which gives priority to impairments, physical and/or intellectual, as being the cause of disability (Rieser and Mason 1990). In this brief attempt to highlight some of the unacceptable features of this approach, it must not be assumed that disabled people do not need, or see, at specific points in their lives, the necessity of medical support. What is being challenged are the social conditions and relations in which such encounters take place, the enveloping their identity in medical terms, the importance of their voice being heard and a much more effective participation in decisions which affect them.

One of the dangers we face today is a possible loss of collective memory (Apple 1993). So much is happening in the present to capture our attention that the necessity and advantages of a historically informed understanding of the past is being lost. As sociologists we are interested in issues of continuity and change. In relation to disability, questions of power, justice, equality, citizenship and participatory democracy are significant issues. How key ideas have been conceived in the past, by whom, under what conditions, and with what consequences are topics worthy of careful sociological exploration. What we experience today, who we are, have their roots in the past. If we are to guard against the excess faddishness of some contemporary perspectives and the regressive relativism of particular forms of postmodernism, and develop a sound basis for future developments, then we do need more historically based sociological studies. The benefits of historical understanding are one of the essential preconditions of an effective struggle for change. Indeed, one of the serious weaknesses of much of the material on empowerment or emancipation is its lack of any historical grounding or political realism. Thus in Giddens' terms, what sociology needs, and particularly in relation to disability, is a strong historical sensibility.

Another gap requiring more sociological work concerns the politics of difference. The disability movement has begun to

be analysed in terms of a new social movement in modern
societies (Oliver 1990; Shakespeare 1993). This includes the
question of collective solidarity. Particular criticisms have been
made concerning the degree to which people with learning
difficulties, gay and lesbian disabled people and disabled women
are adequately represented and feel part of the movement
(Morris 1991). Thus, for example, the degree of marginalisation
is intensified in the lives of disabled women, as Begum, a disabled
black woman, so powerfully reminds us:

Disabled women have become perennial outsiders, our powerless
position has not been seriously addressed by either the disability rights
or the women's movement. The simultaneous neglect is unforgivable.

(1992:73)

Disabled women mediate their experiences within gendered
relations. These compound the oppressions involved. This results
in differences in perception and understanding. Oppression
involves relations of domination and the absence of choices
in the lives of the oppressed (Hooks 1984). Disability, like
race, is part of an overarching structure of domination. This
involves a rejection of an additive approach to oppression in
favour of an interlocking perspective (Hill-Collins 1991). How
we see oppressed groups *relationally* is of central importance.
Challenging disabilist oppression is a necessary step in the struggle
to eradicate *all* forms of oppression.

Drawing on the writings of the black feminist Avtah Brah (1991)
I want to argue for the importance of the distinction between
a notion of 'difference' which emphasises the distinctiveness of
collective histories and thus is concerned with structural conditions
and social relations and that which conceives difference in terms
of experiential diversity. Thus, consideration needs to be given
to identifying the ways in which oppression is structured and
legitimated in the taken-for-granted norms, habits and rules of
institutions. This is part of the systematic constraints operating
on oppressed groups. Complementing such concerns will be the
need to explore the ways in which identities are constructed in
multiple and contradictory ways. The significance of such work
is contingent upon the recognition that the meaning of difference
is a terrain of political struggle (Young 1990). Assimilation and
accommodation theories are being rejected here for a vision of
the good society in which group difference is not eliminated or
transcended, but rather, as Young (1990) contends:

There is equality among socially and culturally differentiated groups,
who mutually respect one another and affirm one another in their
difference.

(1990:63)

Much more sociological work needs to be undertaken in relation to these issues including the exploration of the value of the notion of 'simultaneous oppression' (Stuart 1992). What does it mean, for example, to be disabled, black and a woman?

The struggle of disabled people is against discrimination and prejudice as it is expressed in individual and institutional forms. This essential but difficult task is as Shakespeare notes, for example:

about the 'victim' refusing that label, and instead focusing attention on the structural causes of victimisation. It is about the subversion of stigma: taking a negative appellation and converting it into a badge of pride.

(1993:253)

Disabled people are thus involved, in varying degrees of intensity and effectiveness, in a struggle to capture the power of naming difference itself. An emancipatory meaning of difference is one of the goals of social justice. This entails challenging definitions which isolate and marginalise and replacing them with those which engender solidarity and dignity.

This is part of the endeavour for effective participatic . in society on the part of disabled people which involves challenging the existing power relations and conditions as well as developing a positive self-identity. Johnny Crescendo, the disabled singer, has captured these concerns in the following vivid way:

It's about being comfortable in who you are as a disabled person. It's about having the self respect and the self confidence to challenge the system that screws me and you . . . There's a war goin' on for our right to be included in the human race. Stay Strong. Stay Proud. Stay Angry. GET INVOLVED.

(Cassette – entitled PRIDE)

Thus there is a refusal to accept the deficit and dependency role which has powerfully shaped policies and practices. The language used to describe these endeavours is that of a war, struggle, a battle. The use of such discourse reminds us of the stubbornness and pervasiveness of that which is being opposed. It highlights the degree of commitment required by those engaged in such efforts. It reinforces the social and political nature of the task and the importance of collective solidarity. Finally, it assumes that there are no easy, quick answers to what are fundamentally complex and often contradictory issues.

These sentiments are reflected by Barnes, a disabled analyst, in a powerful statement in which he maintains that:

The abolition of institutional discrimination against disabled people is *not* a marginal activity; it strikes at the heart of social organisations within both the public and private sectors. It would not be possible to confront this problem without being involved in political debate and taking up positions on a wide range of issues [my emphasis].

(1991:233)

In an analysis of social policy in the past decade Glendinning argues that the case of disabled people has actually got *worse* in that:

The economic and social policies of the last decade have done little to enhance, and much to damage, the quality of life of disabled people. Despite the rhetoric of 'protecting' the most 'deserving', 'vulnerable', or 'needy', much of this 'protection' has been illusory.

(1991:16)

These events have culminated in a serious reduction in the degree of autonomy and choice of disabled people and an increase and intensification of 'scrutiny and control by professionals and others' (p. 16).

Projects undertaken since this serious criticism was made continue to reinforce such concerns. For example, in a project examining the extent to which community care can promote independent living for disabled people, Morris (1993) interviewed disabled people, all of whom required assistance in daily living tasks. Several consistent findings confirmed the sense of hopelessness and helplessness that many disabled people experience when trying to get access to statutory services. These services were often not able to respond to the particular or changing requirements of disabled people. The ideology of 'caring' for someone which underpins practice in the social and health services predominantly means 'taking responsibility for them, taking charge of them' (Morris 1993:38). This necessarily involves relations of dependence and an emphasis on 'fitting the client to the service' (p. 20). These factors contributed to a custodial notion of caring. Too often statutory services were based on the assumption that 'physical impairment is the barrier to asserting choice and control' (p. 42) rather than how it is responded to. In another research project Bewley and Glendinning (1994) explored how far disabled people are consulted about the preparation of Community Care Plans. The research included a survey of Community Care Plans in LEAs in England and Wales and detailed studies of a number of authorities. Some of the main findings revealed that very little energy and resources have gone into the production of appropriate materials for people with learning difficulties. Many disabled people gave examples of how they had been effectively excluded by the format of the meetings, the predominance of paperwork, technical terminology, professional jargon and the shared understandings of social services staff. Thus, there was little opportunity for disabled people to define those issues relating to Community Care which they thought were important. Finally, there was a clear failure to recognise the unequal power relations between those who control the provision of services and the disabled people for whom these services are essential to maintain their personal independence.

Disabled people, both individually and through their organisations, have been campaigning for a range of changes with such professional bodies. These include demands for greater choice in the nature and amount of services provided, more control over allocations of resources, especially in relation to independent living, and new forms of accountability of service providers to disabled people involving clear mechanisms for handling disagreements (Brisenden 1986; Oliver and Hasler 1987; Finkelstein 1995).

Conclusion

To be disabled means to be discriminated against. It involves social isolation and restriction. Disability is a significant means of social differentiation in modern societies. The level of esteem and the social standing of disabled people is derived from their position in relation to the wider social conditions and relations of a given society (The Equality Studies Centre 1994; Finkelstein 1995).

Particular institutions can have a significant influence on social status. Status is influenced by the cultural images which, for example, the media portray of particular groups, as well as the legal rights and protection offered them (Barnes & Oliver 1995; Corbett & Ralph 1995). How a society excludes particular groups or individuals involves processes of categorisation in which the inabilities, and the unacceptable and inferior aspects of a person are generated and legitimated.

Disabled people are increasingly involved in challenging such stereotypes and developing an alternative dignified perspective, one which recognises disability as a human rights issue. This involves the struggle for choice, social justice and participation. The voices of disabled people are unmistakably clear on these issues. Listen to these:

In a sense it is startlingly simple. We live in a world which depends for its smooth functioning on marginalising all those for whom its living, working and leisure space was not designed. But we are not just marginalised, we are oppressed and the oppression and abuse have one central identical effect – to make the victims blame themselves and feel that they are bad.

(Cross 1994:164)

or again

> Our vision is of a society which recognises our rights and our value as equal citizens rather than merely treating us as the recipient of other people's goodwill.
>
> (Morris 1992:10)

This commitment to human rights is based on the belief that the world is changeable and that we need to find effective ways of struggling to get things changed (Richardson 1991).

Part of this struggle must be concerned with establishing a public confirmation that discrimination against disabled people is not acceptable. This will require anti-discrimination legislation and political action. In a book entitled *Meeting Disability: A European Response*, Daunt 'explores the intersection between the political integration of Europe and the social integration of disabled people'. He also maintains that:

> . . . . everything we do in relation to disability should be founded on two complementary principles . . . .
> 1.   The principle that all measures should be founded on the explicit recognition of the *rights* of disabled people.
> 2.   The principle that all people are to be regarded as of *equal* value in the society and to the society.
>
> (1991:184)

The extent to which we recognise the value of such principles and seek to implement them in our everyday lives will be contingent upon the degree to which we recognise the profound seriousness of the oppression of disabled people.

In this chapter there has been an encouragement to develop a self-critical approach to the sociological engagement with the issue of disability. An adequate sociology of disability will entail an exploration of issues of power, social justice, citizenship and human rights. Ultimately, fundamental questions need to be asked about the current structural and social conditions and relations of society and how these in complex, and often contradictory ways, establish and legitimate the creation of barriers. The economic, material and ideological forces involved need to be challenged and changed if institutional discrimination is to be overcome.

The issue of disability raises difficult questions that are not only to be examined and engaged with at a societal or policy level, but also at an individual one. What vision do you have with regard to your society and to what extent is your concern over the question of disability inspired by a human rights approach? An important way to begin to seriously engage with such questions is to listen to the voices of disabled people as they are expressed, for example, through their writings, songs and plays.

References

Abberley, P. (1987) 'The concept of oppression and the development of a social theory of disability' in *Disability, Handicap & Society*, Vol. 2, No. 1, pp. 5–20.

Abberley, P. (1992) 'Counting us out: A discussion of the OPCS disability surveys' in *Disability, Handicap & Society*, Vol. 7, No. 2, pp. 139–56.

Acker, S., Barry, K. & Esseveld, J. (1983) 'Objectivity & truth: problems in doing feminist research' in *Women's Studies International Forum* 6, pp. 423–35.

Apple, M. (1993) 'What postmodernists forget: cultural capital and official knowledge' in *Curriculum Studies*, Vol. 1, No. 3, pp. 301–16.

Barbalet, J. (1993) 'Citizenship, class inequality and resentment' in Turner, B. (Ed.) *Citizenship & Social Theory*. London: Sage.

Barnes, C. (1991) *Disabled People in Britain and Discrimination. A Case for Anti-discrimination Legislation*. London: Hurst & Company.

Barnes, C. & Oliver, M. (1995) 'Disability rights: rhetoric and reality in the UK' in *Disability & Society*, Vol. 10, No. 1, pp. 111–16.

Barton, L. & Oliver, M. (1992) 'Special needs: personal trouble or public issue?' in Arnot, M. & Barton, L. (Eds.) *Voicing Concerns. Sociological Perspectives on Contemporary Education Reform*. Wallingford: Triangle Books.

Barton, L. & Tomlinson, S. (Eds.) (1981) *Special Education: Policy, Practices and Social Issues*. London: Harper & Row.

Barton, L. & Tomlinson, S. (Eds.) (1984) *Special Education and Social Interests*. Beckenham: Croom Helm.

Begum, N. (1992) 'Disabled women and the feminist agenda' in *Feminist Review*, No. 40, pp. 70–84.

Bewley, C. & Glendinning, C. (1994) 'Representing the views of disabled people in community care planning', in *Disability & Society* (Special Issue) Vol. 9, No. 3, pp. 301–14.

Bines, H. (1986) *Redefining Remedial Education*. Beckenham: Croom Helm.

Brah, A. (1991) 'Questions of difference and international feminism' in Aaron, J. & Walby, S. (Eds.) *Out of the Margins. Women's Studies in the Nineties*. Lewes: Falmer Press.

Brisenden, S. (1986) Independent living and the medical model of disability in *Disability, Handicap & Society*, Vol. 1, No. 2, pp. 173–8.

Corbett, J. & Ralph, S. (1995) 'The changing image of charity advertising: a case study of Mencap'. Paper presented at The Fourth International Special Education Congress, Birmingham, UK 10–13 April.

Connell, R. (1993) *Schools and Social Justice*. Philadelphia: Temple University Press.

Crescendo, J. (1993) *Pride*. A song on the cassette Pride.

Cross, M. (1994) 'Abuse' in Keith, L. (Ed.) *Mustn't Grumble*. London: The Women's Press.

Daunt, P. (1991) *Meeting Disability: A European Response*. London: Cassell.

Finkelstein, V. (1995) *'Disabling Society: Enabling Interventions. Workbook 4'*. K255 The Disabling Society. Open University; School of Health, Welfare and Community Education.

Fulcher, G. (1989) *Disabling Policies? A Comparative Approach to Education Policy and Disability*. Lewes: Falmer Press.

Giddens, A. (1986) *Sociology. A Brief Critical Introduction*. London: Macmillan. (Second Edition).

Giddens, A. (1991) *Modernity and Self Identity. Self and Society in the Late Modern Age*. Cambridge: Polity Press.

Glendinning, C. (1991) 'Losing ground: social policy and disabled people in Great Britain 1980–90' *Disability, Handicap & Society*, Vol. 6, No. 1, pp. 3–20.

Hahn, H. (1986) Public support for rehabilitation programs: the analysis of US Disability Policy, in *Disability, Handicap & Society*, Vol. 1, No. 2, pp. 121–38.

Hahn, H. (1993) 'The potential impact of disability studies on political science (as well as vice-versa)' in *Policy Studies Journal*, Vol. 21, No. 4, pp. 740–51.

Harvey, L. (1990) *Critical Social Research*. London: Allen & Unwin.

Hill-Collins, P. (1991) *Black Feminist Thought*. London: Routledge.

Hooks, B. (1984) *Feminist Theory from Margin to Centre*. Boston: South End Press.

Jenkins, R. (1991) 'Disability and social stratification' *British Journal of Sociology*, Vol. 42, No. 4, pp. 557–80.

Mills, C. W. (1970) *The Sociological Imagination*. Harmondsworth: Penguin.

Morris, J. (1991) *Pride against Prejudice: Transferring Attitudes to Disability*. London: Women's Press.

Morris, J. (1992a) Quoted in Jones, L. & Pullen, G. 'Cultural differences: deaf and hearing researchers working together' *Disability, Handicap & Society*, Vol. 7, No. 2, pp. 189–96 (Special Issue).

Morris, J. (1992b) *Disabled Lives. Many Voices, One Message*. London: BBC.

Morris, J. (1993) *Community Care or Independent Living*. York: Joseph Rowntree Foundation.

Oliver, M. & Hasler, F. (1987) 'Disability and self-help: A case study of the Spinal Injuries Association' *Disability, Handicap & Society*, Vol. 2, No. 2, pp. 113–25.

Oliver, M. (1989) *Disability and dependency: A creation of Industrial Societies* in Barton, L. (Ed.) *Disability and Dependency*. Lewes: Falmer Press.

Oliver, M. (1990) *The Politics of Disablement*. Basingstoke: Macmillan.

Oliver, M. (1992) 'Changing the social relations of research production?' *Disability, Handicap & Society*, Vol. 7, No. 2, pp. 101–14 (Special Issue).

Quicke, J. (1986) 'A case of paradigmatic mentality? a reply to Mike Oliver' *British Journal of Sociology of Education*, Vol. 7, No. 1, pp. 81–6.

Rieser, R. & Mason, M. (Eds.) (1990) *Disability, Equality in the Classroom: A Human Rights Issue*. London: ILEA.

Richardson, R. (1991) 'Introduction: a visitor yet a part of everybody – the tasks and goals of human rights education' in Starkey, H. (Ed.) *The Challenge of Human Rights Education*. London: Cassell.

Ryan, J. & Thomas, F. (1980) *The Politics of Mental Handicap*. Harmondsworth: Penguin.

Shakespeare, T. (1993) 'Disabled people's self organisation: a new social movement?' in *Disability, Handicap & Society*, Vol. 8, No. 3, pp. 249–64 (Special Issue).

Stuart, O. (1992) 'Race and disability: just a double oppression?' in *Disability, Handicap & Society*, Vol. 7, No. 2, pp. 177–88.

The Equality Studies Centre (1994) *'Equality, Status and Disability'*. Dublin: University College Dublin.

Tomlinson, S. (1982) *The Sociology of Special Education*. London: Routledge & Kegan Paul.

Troyna, B. (1994) 'Blind faith? "empowerment" and educational research' in *International Studies in Sociology of Education*, Vol. 4, No. 1, pp. 3–24.

Young, I. (1990) *Justice and the Politics of Difference*. New Jersey: Princeton University Press.

CHAPTER 2

A sociology of disability or a disablist sociology?

MIKE OLIVER

This chapter will attempt to sketch out the relationship between the enterprise of sociology and the emergence of theorising about disability. It will provide a framework to audit the state of that relationship and suggest ways in which the relationship might develop in the future. In so doing it will concentrate on British and American sociology and work done on physical impairment. Space does not permit that theoretical developments from Australia and Canada in particular nor that work on the sociology of learning difficulty and sensory impairment can be incorporated. Important work on the sociology of special education has also been omitted for this reason.

Sociology and disability theory: a case for concern

Elsewhere in this volume Barton discusses the relationship between sociology and disability in more detail and is critical of sociology's lack of interest in disability issues. I don't wish to reproduce my version of that discussion here but to point out that Barton refers to the work of Giddens (1986; 1991) in his comments. Undoubtedly, the leading British sociologist of his generation, Giddens has produced one of the most popular introductory sociology texts (1989) and in it, there is not a single mention of disability; close examination of many other introductory texts will yield similar results.

This, of course, is not proof of the thesis that sociology has ignored disability completely but is testament to the fact that disability has hardly figured at all on the sociological agenda. The major reasons for this have been that disability has been regarded as both a medical issue and an individual problem. Hence it is to the disciplines of medicine and psychology that disability has been confined as an object of theoretical and empirical concern.

Even where disability would be expected to be part of the 'sociological turf', as in medical sociology, the discipline and its practitioners have often failed to challenge the individualisation and medicalisation of disability. Recently, a number of sociologists working in the general area of medical sociology and chronic illness have expressed concern over the growing importance of the 'social oppression theory' of disability, its associated research methodologies, and their implications for doing research in the 'chronic illness and disability fields' (Bury 1992).

Stemming from the influence of Foucault, sociology has recently rekindled its interest in the body, an area where it might reasonably be expected that 'the disabled body' could be central to any theoretical or conceptual innovations. However, sociologists working in this area reproduce the disablism that sociology exhibits everywhere else; sociologists of the body either ignore disability completely or they analyse it as if it were the same phenomenon as illness.

Hence a recent collection on the topic (Featherstone, Hepworth and Turner 1991) virtually ignores disability except for one article by Arthur Frank. In his analytical review, he provides his own typology which virtually ignores disability, explaining his reason thus;

It is not a condition which fits my diagram, thus demonstrating that any theory must have its residual categories.

(Frank 1991:87)

So disabled people are not only relegated to the margins of society, they are relegated to the margins of sociological theory as well.

From the margins several sociologists have taken disability seriously; the following two sections will attempt to briefly describe this, focusing initially on American sociology before moving to talk about Britain. Separating the two traditions in this way will mean that some of the interconnections between the two may not be given enough attention; as, for example, with the undoubted influence of American sociological theorists such as Parsons, Becker and Goffman on medical sociology in Britain.

Sociological accounts of disability

Like mainstream American sociology itself, American sociology of disability has been profoundly influenced by functionalist and interactionist theories. It is this influence that we will consider here.

Much American sociological writing on disability is rooted in the work of Parsons and his analysis of sickness-related behaviour. This is because the Parsonian paradigm has been principally responsible for two distinct, but interdependent, approaches which have implicitly or explicitly influenced all subsequent analyses. They are the relevance of the 'sick role' in relation to disability and its association with social deviance, and the notion of health as adaptation (Bury 1982).

Briefly, Parsons' (1951) model suggests that at the onset of illness 'sick' people should adopt the sick role. Rooted in the assumption that illness and disease impede both physiological and psychological abilities, 'sick' individuals are automatically relieved of all normal expectations and responsibilities. Generally considered unaccountable for their condition, they are not expected to recover through their own volition. They are encouraged to view their present situation as 'abhorrent and undesirable', and, in order to regain their former status, are expected to seek help from professional medical experts (Parsons 1951).

Parsons' model assumes that regardless of the nature of the condition or the socio-economic factors involved everyone will behave in exactly the same way. It pays little heed to subjective interpretation and articulates only the views of the representatives of society credited with the responsibility for recovery, i.e. the medical profession. It does not accommodate sick role variation (Twaddle 1969) nor the distinction between illness and impairment (Gordon 1966; Sieglar & Osmond 1974).

Occupation of the sick role is intended to be temporary. But the same assumptions are applied to people with impairments. The 'impaired role', for example, is ascribed to an individual whose condition is unlikely to change and who is unable or unwilling to meet the first prerequisite of the sick role; to 'get well' as quickly as possible. Occupants of this construct are said to have abandoned the idea of recovery altogether and accepted dependency. Signifying a loss of 'full human status' the impaired role does 'not require the exertions of cooperating with medical treatment and trying to regain one's health, but the price for this is a kind of second-class citizenship' (Sieglar & Osmond 1974:116).

A further variation on this train of thought is the 'rehabilitation role' as articulated by Safilios-Rothschild (1970). This model suggests that once a person with an impairment becomes aware of their condition they must accept it and learn how to live with it. This is achieved, it is argued, through the maximisation of existing abilities. Within this frame of reference individuals with impairments are obligated to assume as many 'normal' functions as they can, as quickly as possible. They are not exempt from social expectations or responsibilities but must adapt accordingly. Additionally, they should cooperate with professionals and innovate and ameliorate new methods of rehabilitation.

Clearly, the locus of responsibility rests squarely on the shoulders of the person with an impairment. They are dependent upon the rehabilitation professionals for at least two specific functions; first, the initiation of rehabilitation programmes designed to return individuals with impairments to 'normality', and, second, assistance in the psychological accommodation of a 'disabled' identity. The process of cognitive adjustment to impairment is usually presented as a series of psychological stages such as 'shock', 'denial', 'anger' and 'depression'. Movement is sequential and generally seen as only one way. Passage through each stage is determined by an acceptable time frame according to professionally agreed criteria (Albrecht 1976).

Apart from the fact that there is substantial evidence questioning the empirical validity of these theories (Silver and Wortman 1980) they can be criticised on at least three different levels. First, they are essentially determinist; behaviour is only viewed positively if it is commensurate with professionals' perceptions of reality. Second, they ignore extraneous economic, political and social factors. Third, they undermine and deny subjective interpretations of impairment from the perspective of the person concerned.

In short, they are the product of the 'psychological imagination' constructed upon a bedrock of 'non-disabled' assumptions of what it is like to experience impairment (Oliver 1983). The realisation of impairment is presumed to involve some form of loss or 'personal tragedy'. Thus, this individualistic medical approach can best be understood as 'personal tragedy theory' (Oliver 1986).

One important factor explaining the continued ideological hegemony of 'personal tragedy theory' is its professional expediency, both at the individual and at the structural levels. If individuals fail to achieve the anticipated professionally determined rehabilitation goals then this failure can be explained with reference to the disabled person's perceived inadequacy – whether it be physically or intellectually based or both. The 'expert' is exonerated from responsibility, professional integrity remains intact, traditional wisdom and values are not questioned, and the existing social order remains unchallenged (Barnes 1990).

Interactionist theory has conceptualised disability as social deviance and suggests that the relationship between disability and deviance can be understood with reference to the freedom from social obligations and responsibilities explicit in the sick role construct and in the negative view of impairment prevalent in industrial and post-industrial societies. Because such societies are founded upon liberal ideals of individual responsibility, competition and paid employment, those who are perceived to be unable to meet these ideals are regarded as deviant.

The analysis of social reaction toward disadvantaged minority groups, such as people with impairments, was central for sociologists working within the traditions of symbolic inter-actionism during the 1960s. Emphasising meaning, identity and the process of labelling, they explored the relationship between disablement and socially proscribed behaviour. Initially, sociologists working within this perspective were interested in crime and drug addiction but, following substantial ethnographic research, they turned their attention towards the mechanisms of deviance creation and the labelling process (Becker 1963).

Lemert (1962) made the distinction between 'primary' and 'secondary' deviance; the former having only marginal impli-cations for the individual concerned and the latter relating to the ascription by others of a socially devalued status and identity. Secondary deviance becomes a central facet of existence for those so labelled, 'altering psychic structure' producing specialised social roles for self-management. Lemert (1962) discusses disability extensively but, like Parsonian sociology, fails to treat illness and disability as conceptually distinct.

Goffman (1963) developed interactionist theory further with his use of the concept 'stigma', a term, he claimed, was used traditionally to refer to a mark or blemish denoting 'moral inferiority' necessitating avoidance by the rest of society. He suggested that the 'stigmatised' such as 'the dwarf, the blind man, the disfigured . . ., and the ex-mental patient' are generally viewed as not quite human. For Goffman, the application of stigma is the outcome of situational considerations and social interactions between the 'normal' and the 'abnormal'.

Clearly, Goffman's use of the term 'stigma' is based upon perceptions of the oppressor rather than those of the oppressed. Derived from the Greek practice of marking slaves, the appli-cation of stigma is an issue of exploitation and oppression rather than avoidance; slave masters did not avoid their slaves – they used and abused them for their most personal, intimate and sexual needs.

In the modern context Goffman fails to move beyond the individual with his focus on the discredited and discreditable; takes as given the imposed segregation, passivity and inferior status of stigmatised individuals and groups – including disabled people – ingrained in capitalist social relations, without seriously addressing questions of causality (Finkelstein 1980). Davis (1964) reproduces this failure and also fails to move beyond personal tragedy theory in his study of polio *victims* (my emphasis), conceptualising the responses of his subjects as disavowal rather than resistance.

As a consequence, while some sociologists have seen stigma as the way forward in understanding disability (e.g. Ainley *et al.* 1986), disabled people have preferred to reinterpret their collective experiences in terms of structural notions of discrimination and oppression rather than interpersonal ones of stigma and stigmatisation.

(Oliver 1990:68)

By the late 1960s the dominance of functionalism and inter-actionism within American sociology was being questioned (Gouldner 1971; 1975), if not challenged. It was at this point that two texts specifically on disability were published which provided a synthesis of these two dominant traditions. Scott's (1969) cross-national study of blindness featured both functionalism in its use of the central values of a range of societies and interactionism in its exploration of the ways these values shaped the experience of blindness. Safilios-Rothschild's (1970) text was a theoretical synthesis of the two traditions and also opened up the sociology of disability towards the conflict approaches which were beginning to emerge in American sociology generally.

It was at this point that the struggles of disabled people in North America for independent living and civil rights were beginning to make an impact. The analysis of these collective struggles was easier within the newly emerging conflict sociology. These struggles to achieve independent living (De Jong 1979) through ending discrimination and articulating their rights to be included in society has led to the emergence of a 'socio-political' approach in American sociology. In the forefront of this approach, just as in Britain, have been disabled people themselves, such as Hahn (1988) and Zola (1979).

Disabled women too, have begun to articulate their concerns and to use feminist sociology as a tool to do this (Deegan and Brooks 1985). The links between the academic community and disabled people has begun to be established with the founding of The Society for Disability Studies and the publication of its journal *Disability Quarterly*.

While in some ways then, the relationship between American sociology and disability is therefore more developed than it is in Britain, it has still been unable to shake off the legacy of functionalism and interactionism with its consensual under-pinnings and the fact that, twenty years on, American conflict sociology has remained essentially pluralist.

A recent book by a leading American sociologist of disability (Albrecht 1992), for example, claims 'to provide a new perspective to the study of disability and rehabilitation' and the publisher's blurb further claims that the book presents 'a fresh, new metaphor to help recast our understanding of disability and the rehabilitation industry'.

Central to the claim of a new perspective is the idea that disability is produced: as distinct from it simply being some medical or physiological abnormality; as distinct from it being socially constructed as deviance; as distinct from the arguments of disabled people that they are a minority group.

A person's position in society affects the type and severity of physical disability one is likely to experience and more importantly the likelihood that he or she is likely to receive rehabilitation services. Indeed, the political economy of a community dictates what debilitating health conditions will be produced, how and under what circumstances they will be defined, and ultimately who will receive the services.

(Albrecht 1992:14)

However, the structure of capitalist America itself goes unexamined. Certainly the book mentions the fact that issues like poverty, race, gender and age are factors in the production of disability, but the centrality of these issues to both theoretical and experiential understandings of disability is never acknowledged, nor is the important work being undertaken in advancing these perspectives by disabled women and black disabled people.

Similarly, post-modernism merits a mention but nowhere is it discussed nor its impact on the production of disability analysed. In fact, Albrecht's concept of post-modernism can be reduced to a mention of the coming of new technologies and the rise of service industries and professionals. Again this issue is serious because without a properly theorised conception of post-modernity, it is difficult to understand recent work around the cultural production and representation of disability. Indeed, it is clear that Albrecht's arguments have been unable to shake off the shackles of functionalism and interactionism, such as when he makes statements like:

Persons with disabilities must either accept the socially constructed definition laid on them or fight for a personal redefinition.

(Albrecht 1992:275)

This lack of understanding is compounded when discussing the disability movement almost exclusively in terms of advocacy and self-help. Again no mention of the significance of new social movements in general and the disability movement in particular, and the real challenge they pose to the production of disability, its cultural representations and the possible transformation of rehabilitation from a commodity to a political weapon.

In the end, Albrecht may eschew interactionist and functionalist sociology in claiming to produce something new, but when he comments that

The challenge is to create a social policy and realistic programs based upon the existing political economy of the rehabilitation business that serves the needs of all persons with disabilities.

(Albrecht 1992:317)

it is clear that pluralism, in either its conflict or consensus variants, still rules American sociology.

Accounts of disablist sociology

In Britain, as I have already suggested, sociology has paid little attention to the issue of disability, although medical sociology has forayed into the area on occasions in the past (Blaxter 1976; Locker 1985) and more recently (Scambler 1989; Robinson 1988). In addition, sociologists like Walker and Townsend (1981) have used Fabian policy analysis to discuss disability in the context of poverty and inequality.

None of this work, however, has been located within the critical or emancipatory projects that have accompanied some sociological theorising. In this section, I want to trace the emergence of a critical and emancipatory sociology as it has emerged within the British sociological tradition.

We can trace a gradually awakening of sociological interest in the area, stemming almost exclusively from the ideas of disabled people themselves, many of whom were not sociologists. In 1966 a collection of essays written by disabled people appeared (Hunt 1966). The final essay in the piece by Paul Hunt was a critical analysis of the role of disabled people in society written from a radical rather than a functionalist position. Another essay in the collection by Louis Battye could be said to be the forerunner of later important work on cultural representation by people like Hevey (1992), Shakespeare (1993) and Darke (1994).

Paul Hunt was influential not only through his writings. He also became a key participant in the Union of the Physically Impaired Against Segregation (UPIAS). This was a newly formed collective of disabled people who, after meeting regularly to share their experiences and further their personal struggles collectively, came to the conclusion that disability was a form of social oppression.

In our view, it is society which disables physically impaired people. Disability is something imposed on top of our impairments by the way we are unnecessarily isolated and excluded from full participation in society. Disabled people are therefore an oppressed group in society. To understand this it is necessary to grasp the distinction between the physical impairment and the social situation, called 'disability', of people with such impairment. Thus we define impairment as lacking part of or all of a limb, or having a defective limb, organ or mechanism of the body; and disability as the disadvantage or restriction of activity caused by a contemporary social organisation which takes no or little account of people who have physical impairments and thus excludes them from participation in the mainstream of social activities. Physical disability is therefore a particular form of social oppression.

(UPIAS 1976:3–4)

It seemed at the time of the publication of *Fundamental Principles of Disability* that the sociological imagination, at least as far as disability was concerned, was being exercised by non-sociologists. The next step in the sociological history of disability was also taken by a non-sociologist. In 1980 Finkelstein, who had trained as a psychologist and was also active in UPIAS, published his pathbreaking *Attitudes and Disabled People* in which he outlined a materialist approach to our understanding of disability, arguing that disability was a relationship mediated by the interactions between economic and social structures and individual impairment.

Both of these publications profoundly influenced my own writing and led to my identification of 'the social model of disability' (Oliver 1983) which became the central concept around which disabled people began to interpret their own experiences and organise their own political movement. The next major step came with the founding of the international journal, then called *Disability, Handicap and Society*, first published in 1986. While not exclusively a sociology journal, it was the first journal to take the issue of social theorising in respect of disability seriously.

It was Abberley's (1987) paper in this journal which was to take the idea of disability as oppression much further than UPIAS had done, placing it in a sociological context and introducing the concept of disablism alongside those of racism and sexism. His conclusion was an unwelcome although accurate depiction of the disablism inherent in the sociological enterprise.

the sociology of disability is both theoretically backward and a hindrance rather than a help to disabled people. In particular it has ignored the implications of significant advances made in the last 15 years in the study of sexual and racial inequality, and reproduces in the study of disability parallel deficiencies to those found in what is now seen by many as racist and sexist sociology. Another aspect of 'good sociology' that I feel is generally absent is any significant recognition of the historical specificity of the experience of disability.

(Abberley 1987:5)

The next significant advance was the publication of my own materialist account of the production of disability as a medicalised and individualised condition within the social relations of capitalist production (Oliver 1990), of which more will be said in the next section. This was partly an attempt to take further Finkelstein's earlier materialist account of disability. More so, it was an attempt to apply my own sociological imagination to both my own personal experiences as a disabled person and to make sense of the political and social changes that were beginning to occur as a result of disabled people's attempts at collective self-organisation.

The following year produced two further significant advances. Firstly there was the publication of Barnes's *Disabled People in Britain and Discrimination* (1991) which introduced the idea of institutionalised discrimination against disabled people, documented its pervasiveness throughout British society and made a passionate plea for anti-discrimination legislation. Secondly, Morris (1991) produced a feminist account of the experience of disability which was both a critique of earlier, male-dominated sociological accounts of disability as well as being a celebration of the lives of disabled women.

The next major advance was the publication of a special edition of *Disability, Handicap and Society* (Vol. 7, No. 2, 1992) devoted to disability research. It raised important questions about both the positivist and interpretive research paradigms and introduced new concepts and issues onto the sociological agenda. It challenged existing social relations of research production, questioned previous accounts of the lives of disabled people through introducing the concept of simultaneous oppression and suggested ways in which research on disability issues should struggle against being oppressive and disablist.

Hevey's (1992) sustained attack on charities was the next publication of importance as far as the sociological agenda is concerned. As well as being an analysis of the organisation and operation of charitable organisations, it also produced a sophisticated theoretical examination of the cultural representation of disabled people through tragic imagery. While it may not have quite been post-modernist sociological theory, it was very close to it.

The work of Shakespeare (1993; 1994a) is more clearly influenced by post-modernist ideas. He contends that not only do disabled people face the problems of discrimination engendered by the material relations of production but also the problems of prejudice engendered by cultural representations of disabled people as 'other' throughout history.

I have shifted away from attempts to construct over-arching theoretical models, or to impose rational structures on the experiences of disability, towards an approach which stresses subjectivity; the contingency, conflict and discontinuity within the disability experience and individual disabled identities. To a certain extent, I have moved closer to post-modern sociological approaches . . .

(Shakespeare 1994b:195)

It is at this intersection between materialist, feminist and post-modernist theorising that the sociological imagination has arrived; at least it has for those few sociologists and others currently working in the area. Speculation about where we might go from here will be discussed later; what is needed at present is to provide an audit of where we are now. I shall begin with my own sociological theorising about disability.

Disability and capitalism

Whatever the fate of disabled people before the advent of capitalist society and whatever their fate will be in the brave new world of the 21st century, with its coming we suffered economic and social exclusion. As a consequence of this exclusion disability was produced in a particular form – as an individual problem requiring medical treatment.

The transition to late capitalism (the post-industrial society, as some writers have called it, or its more recent fashionable manifestation as post-modernity) has led to demands for the inclusion of those previously excluded. As a consequence of this, the production of disability as an individual medical problem has increasingly come under attack and attempts to produce disability in a different, social form commensurate with inclusion have been appearing upon the sociological agenda.

The starting point for my own materialist account of disability was the question of whether the medicalised and tragic view of disability that dominated British society was reproduced in other societies. A quick reading of both history and anthropology soon revealed two things. To begin with, it is not only sociology which has failed to take disability seriously, but history and anthropology as well. In addition, what evidence there was showed that the medicalised and tragic view of disability was unique to capitalist societies and other societies viewed disability in a variety of different ways.

Following Finkelstein, and indeed Marx, it seemed fairly clear that the mode of production played a crucial role in that with the rise of capitalism and the coming of individualised wage labour in factories, impaired people were at a severe disadvantage. In fact so many were unable to keep or retain jobs that they became a social problem for the capitalist state whose initial response to all social problems was harsh deterrence and institutionalisation.

Impaired people became a particular problem because they were unable rather than unwilling to cope with the new demands made on the labour force. Hence deterrence was bound to fail and came to be seen as unjust. However, because impaired people could not be integrated into the workforce they still had to be controlled. This was done by providing a range of specialist institutions whose overt aim was to provide treatment or shelter from a harsh world rather than punishment.

This coincided with the rise to prominence of the medical profession who were only too willing to legitimate the categorisation of deserving and undeserving people. As a consequence disabled people became labelled as sick and were placed in a variety of medical institutions. The idea of sickness at this time was that it was a random, unfortunate happening for individuals, giving rise to the idea that impairment was somehow a tragic occurrence that happened to individuals.

As I stated elsewhere, sociology had become very good in penetrating such ideology in areas other than disability, but had not focused its gaze in this particular direction.

A social theory of disability then, should be integrated into, rather than separated from existing social theories. It has to be remembered however, that personal tragedy theory itself has performed a particular ideological function of its own. Like deficit theory as an explanation of poor educational achievement, like sickness as an explanation of criminal behaviour, like character weakness as an explanation of poverty and unemployment, and like all other victim-blaming theories (Ryan, 1971), personal tragedy theory has served to individualise the problems of disability and hence to leave social and economic structures untouched. Social science in general and social policy in particular have progressed far in rejecting individualistic theories and constructing a range of alternative social ones – let us hope that personal tragedy theory, the last in the line, will soon disappear also, to be replaced by a much more adequate social (oppression) theory of disability.

(Oliver 1986:16)

Some ten years later, we have come some way down the road, which is why we need to audit our progress.

Disability production in transition

In order to develop more appropriate sociological accounts of disability, it is necessary to understand that the production of disability is in transition. In this process of transition our complex and difficult task is to understand that this process is one of transition from one world view of disability to another.

This process is what Kuhn (1961) would call a 'paradigm shift' in that the old individualised and medicalised paradigm described in the previous section has so many anomalies that a new paradigm, or indeed a series of paradigms, is in the process of emerging. As yet it is by no means clear what precise shape these new paradigms will take but they are clearly being influenced by materialist, pluralist and post-modernist social theory as well as by the demands of disabled people that their experiences be taken seriously, by sociologists and researchers among others.

There are three basic levels at which we can approach this task of capturing this process of transition of disability paradigms; the ontological, the epistemological and the experiential, see Table 2.1. They lead to the following questions; What is the nature of disability? What causes it? How is it experienced? These basic questions raise different sets of issues at different levels of abstraction.

The ontological level requires issues to be addressed in terms of sociological theory; examples of which we have already discussed

Table 2.1:   **The Hegemony of disability**

Level	Question	Way of understanding
Ontology	What is the nature of disability?	Sociological Theory
Epistemology	What causes disability?	Middle range theories?
Experience	What does it feel like to be disabled?	Methodology

and includes functionalism, interactionism, political economy in both its pluralist and materialist variants. The epistemological level requires issues to be addressed in terms of middle range theorising, the need for which was pointed to in the work of American sociologist Merton (1968). The experiential level requires issues to be addressed in terms of developing an appropriate methodology for understanding the experience of disability from the perspective of disabled people themselves (Campling 1981; Oliver *et al.* 1988; Morris 1989).

These levels do not exist independently of each other except in a conceptual sense. Rather, they interact with each other in producing what might be called the totality, or indeed, the hegemony of disability. Hegemony, as it is used here, describes the ways in which the ontological level, the epistemological and the experiential levels interconnect with each other to form a complete whole.

The hegemony of disability, as it is produced by capitalist society – and it should be re-emphasised that other kinds of society have produced disability in different forms – stems from the ontological assumptions it makes about the pathological and problem-oriented nature of disability.

These ontological assumptions link directly to epistemological concerns about the causes of disability in individuals with a view to eradication through prevention, cure or treatment. Hence the assumption is, in health terms, that disability is pathology and in welfare terms, that disability is a social problem. Treatment, cure and amelioration are the appropriate societal responses to perceived pathologies and problems. Finally these assumptions and concerns exert a considerable influence on the way disability is experienced by both able-bodied and disabled people alike – to have a disability is to have a problem, to have a disability is to have 'something wrong with you'.

In recent years, this hegemony of disability has been under a sustained and persistent attack in late capitalist society. At the ontological level this has led, not to a denial of the problem-oriented nature of disability, but of its assumptions of pathology. At the epistemological level middle-range theorising has been turned on its head; disability is caused not by the functional, physical or psychological limitations of impaired individuals but by the failure of society to remove its disabling barriers and social restrictions. At the experiential level disabled people are increasingly seeing their problems as stemming from social oppression (Sutherland 1981) and institutionalised discrimination (Barnes 1991), leading to the view that impairment is something to celebrate, not cure or ameliorate.

Thus, the argument that the problems of disability are societal rather than individual, and that these problems stem from oppression by society rather than the limitations of individuals, is an essential part of developing an adequate understanding of societal responses to disability. However, in attempting to understand hegemony of disability, the ways in which the individualising of disability is interconnected at the levels of society, policy and practice and personal experience is crucial. These interconnections are crucial to the attempt to reformulate disability as an issue for society and develop a more appropriate social understanding of policy responses, professional practice and personal experience.

At present the individualising and medicalising of disability permeates all three levels and connects them. Disability is seen as a personal tragedy which occurs at random to individuals, and the problems of disability require individuals to adjust or come to terms with this tragedy. Research has used techniques designed to 'prove' the existence of these adjustment problems. The alternative view suggests that disability occurs in structured ways dependent upon the material relations of production (Oliver 1990), the problem of adjustment is one for society, not individuals and that research should be concerned with identifying the ways in which society disables people rather than the effects on individuals (Oliver 1992; Zarb 1992).

Both the current dominant way of understanding disability and alternative formulations are summarised in Table 2.2.

Having provided a diagrammatic summary of the current state of sociology in respect of disability, I want in the remaining sections of this chapter to reflect on my own work in relation to both the old and alternative sociological paradigms.

Sociological theory – personal tragedy, post-modernism or political economy?

Undoubtedly, in terms of the phenomenon of disability, the dominant theory, albeit an implicit one, has been personal tragedy

Table 2.2:   **Old and new paradigms**

Ways of understanding	Old paradigm	Alternatives 1 (Others)	Alternative 2 (Oliver)
Sociological theory	(Personal tragedy)	Socio political	Political economy (materialist)
	Functionalism	Political economy (Pluralist)	
	Interactionism		
		Post-modernism	
Middle-range theorising	Adjustment/loss	Individual rights	Social adjustment
	Sick role	Integration	Inclusion
	Deviance/Stigma	Personal Empowerment	Collective Empowerment
Methodology	Positivist	Participatory	Emancipatory
	Interpretive	Applied Research	
		Action research	

theory. This suggests that disability is a tragic happening that occurs to unfortunate, isolated individuals on a random basis. It further influences compensatory policy responses and therapeutic interventions designed to help individuals come to terms with tragedy. At the level of individual experience, many disabled people come to see their lives as blighted by tragedy.

The problem is that personal tragedy theory does not provide a universalistic explanation of disability; in some societies disability is seen as the ascription of privilege, as a sign of being chosen by the gods. In others it is seen as bringing important social benefits such as bilingualism, as illustrated by the pervasive use of sign language throughout the community that was Martha's Vineyard (Groce 1985). Further, even within some late capitalist societies, policies are moving away from compensation and towards entitlement. Therapeutic interventions are also moving away from adjustment and towards empowerment. Finally, with the developing of a politics of personal identity, the experience of disability is being reinterpreted in positive rather than negative terms (Morris 1991).

The emergence of post-modernism in respect of theorising disability is drawing attention to the important influence of cultural representation in shaping the experience of disability but, in Shakespeare's work, this appears to be reductionist. Barnes elsewhere in this volume suggests that

He rightly suggests that the cultural roots of disabled people's oppression in western society pre-dates the emergence of capitalism. However . . . . he implies that all cultures respond to impairment in essentially negative terms. In other words, prejudice against people with impairments is, in one way or another, inevitable and universal.

(Barnes 1996, Chapter 3 in this volume)

Barnes then goes on to demonstrate, using historical and anthropological evidence, that this is not the case.

Political economy, at least in its materialist variant, suggests that all phenomena (including social categories) are produced by the economic and social forces of capitalism itself. The forms in which they are produced are ultimately dependent upon their relationship to the economy (Marx 1913). Hence, the category disability is produced in the particular form it appears by these very economic and social forces. Further, it is produced as an economic problem because of changes in the nature of work and the needs of the labour market within capitalism.

The speed of factory work, the enforced discipline, the time-keeping and production norms – all these were a highly unfavourable change from the slower, more self-determined methods of work into which many handicapped people had been integrated.

(Ryan & Thomas 1980:101)

Hence the economy, through both the operation of the labour market and the social organisation of work, plays a key role in producing the category disability and in determining societal responses to disabled people. Further, the oppression that disabled people face is rooted in the economic and social structures of capitalism which themselves produce racism, sexism, homophobia, ageism and disablism.

For the vast majority of time throughout the 20th century, work has been organised around the twin principles of competition between individual workers and maximisation of profit. Inevitably disabled people have suffered because of the way work has been organised around those two principles; inevitably we've experienced exclusion from the workforce and even government-commissioned research suggests that at least seven out of ten disabled people who are of working age don't have jobs (Martin, White and Meltzer 1988).

The only time that those figures have substantially changed have been during the two world wars. During the Second World War, 430,000 disabled people who'd previously been excluded from the workforce were incorporated into factories and into industry and not just in menial low-grade tasks, but often doing important supervisory and managerial jobs (Humphreys & Gordon 1992). The reason for that, it seems to me, is absolutely simple. The purpose of work during those two wars was not to maximise profit but to fight the common enemy. Work was organised around the principles of cooperation and collaboration, not around the principles of competition and maximisation of profit.

At the end of the Second World War we saw the election of a government committed to ensuring that the situation continued and they passed legislation to ensure that disabled people were not excluded from the workforce. The reality is that, within three years, not only were most of those disabled people who'd been included into the workforce out of jobs, but most of the other disabled people whose impairments had been created by the War didn't actually get into meaningful employment either. The old principles of the capitalist economy had reasserted themselves.

Hence the political economy perspective suggests that disabled people are excluded from the workforce not because of their personal or functional limitations (old paradigm), nor simply because of discriminatory attitudes and practices among employers and labour markets (alternative 1) but because of the way in which work is organised within the capitalist economy itself (alternative 2).

Middle-range theorising – adjustment and loss or social adjustment?

Middle-range theories are usually concerned to link the abstract concepts of theory to the specific experiences of particular phenomena. So studies of disability within the old paradigm have been dominated by middle-range adjustment theories. These suggest that when something happens to an individual's body something happens to the mind as well. Thus, in order to become fully human again, in order to form a disabled identity, the disabled individual must undergo medical treatment and physical rehabilitation as well as the process of psychological adjustment or coming to terms with disability (Finkelstein 1980).

However, the conceptual framework provided by middle-range adjustment theory has been severely criticised on theoretical grounds (Oliver 1981) as well as on the grounds that it does not accord with the actual experience of disability. Alternative frameworks such as social adjustment (Oliver *et al.* 1988) and social oppression (UPIAS 1976) have been developed.

Within the alternative 1 paradigm, concepts such as individual rights, integration and personal empowerment are prominent. The problem with them, as has already been intimated, is they do not pay sufficient attention to issues of social and economic structure and power. Individuals struggle individually to achieve integration into society as it is and in doing so, empower themselves. It is as if they want the rules of the game to change so that they can play alongside everyone else rather than change the game. The problem, of course, is that if the game is possessive individualism in a competitive and inegalitarian society, impaired people will inevitably be disadvantaged, no matter how the rules are changed.

My own initial work on the long-term effects of spinal cord injury (alternative 2) suggested that the occurrence of a disability as a significant event in an individual's life is only a starting point for understanding the practical and personal consequences of living with disability. The work further suggested that the social environment, material resources and – most importantly – the meanings which individuals attach to situations and events were the most important factors to be considered in developing an adequate conceptual model, which has been called social adjustment.

For us, then, understanding the consequences of spinal cord injury involves a complex relationship between the impaired individual, the social context within which the impairment occurs and the meanings available to individuals to enable them to make sense of what is happening.

(Oliver *et al.* 1988:11)

The experience of spinal cord injury, therefore, cannot be understood in terms of purely internal psychological or inter-personal processes, but requires a whole range of other material factors such as housing, finance, employment, the built environ-ment and family circumstances to be taken into account. Further, all of these material factors can and will change over time, sometimes for the better and sometimes for the worse, hence giving the experience of disability a temporal as well as a material dimension.

Hence the personal responses of individuals to their impair-ments cannot be understood merely as a reaction to trauma or tragedy, nor as a struggle for personal empowerment. Such understandings have to be located in a framework which takes account of disabled people's life histories, their material circumstances and the meaning that disability has for them as they have struggled through collective action to empower themselves and be included in the societies in which they live.

Methodology – describing, interpreting, understanding or changing the experience of disability?

The central methodological issue concerns the purpose of research and whether this is to describe, interpret, understand or change particular phenomena. As far as disability research is concerned, positivistic and interpretive approaches within the old paradigm have been located within the medical model with its in-built assumptions which see disability as individual pathology. Consequently, most of this research is considered to be at best irrelevant, and at worst, oppressive (Oliver 1992).

Even where applied or action approaches have been used, they have failed to change the social relations of research production (Oliver 1992), seeing research as a way of informing policy development or improving professional practice. Lacking in these approaches has been the involvement of disabled people in the research process as active participants rather than passive subjects.

This has resulted in a persistent lack of fit between able-bodied and disabled people's own articulations of their own experience and has had implications for both the provision of services and the ability of individuals to control their own lives. As Davis (1986) points out, research on disability has consistently failed to involve disabled people except as passive objects for interviews and observations designed by researchers with no experience or sensitivity to the day-to-day reality of disability – a situation which, whilst it may be of benefit to researchers, does nothing to serve the interests of disabled people. Thus many disabled people have become alienated from disability research; a not uncommon problem for research subjects, according to one commentator (Rowan 1981).

This disillusion with existing approaches to research has raised the issue of developing an alternative, emancipatory approach in order to make disability research both more relevant to the lives of disabled people and more influential in improving their material circumstances. The two key fundamentals on which such an approach must be based are empowerment and reciprocity. These fundamentals can be built in by encouraging self-reflection and a deeper understanding of the research situation by the research subjects themselves as well as enabling researchers to identify with their research subjects (Lather 1991).

The importance of emancipatory research, therefore,

is in establishing a dialogue between research workers and the grass-roots people with whom they work, in order to discover and realise the practical and cultural needs of those people. Research here becomes one part of a developmental process including also education and political action.

(Reason 1988:2)

Such an understanding is an essential pre-requisite to providing a re-definition of 'the real nature of the problem'. This process has been succinctly captured in a commentary on research on black issues.

It was not black people who should be examined, but white society; it was not a case of educating blacks and whites for integration, but of fighting institutional racism; it was not race relations that was the field for study, but racism.

(Bourne 1980:339)

Ten years later, this quote applies exactly to the 'state' of disability research; it is not disabled people who need to be examined but able-bodied society; it is not a case of educating disabled and able-bodied people for integration, but of fighting institutional disablism; it is not disability relations which should be the field for study but disablism.

But we cannot study disablism, or racism or sexism or any other oppressions in isolation from each other. It has quickly become clear that such notions are over-simplistic and indeed can be oppressive in themselves. As Morris argues:

It is not very helpful to talk about disabled women experiencing a 'double disadvantage'. Images of disadvantage are such an important part of the experience of oppression that emancipatory research (research which seeks to further the interests of 'the researched') must consistently challenge them. Therein lies one of the problems with examining the relationship between gender and disability, race and disability in terms of 'double disadvantage'. The research can itself become part of the oppression.

(Morris 1992:162)

Further, such additive approaches have also been criticised by black disabled people who argue that their experience of disability can only be understood within the context of racism. Thus according to one black researcher,

In my opinion, the concept of double discrimination, as propagated by white disabled feminists is an inadequate framework within which to understand racism within disability . . . on the contrary, I suggest that racism within disability is part of a process of simultaneous oppression which black people experience daily in Western society.

(Stuart 1992:179)

Whether simultaneous oppression offers a more adequate way of understanding disability is something that only further, more developed emancipatory research can show. But certainly people are beginning to talk about their experience in this way.

As a black disabled woman, I cannot compartmentalise or separate aspects of my identity in this way. The collective experience of my race, disability and gender are what shape and inform my life.

(Hill 1994:7)

Whether such a concept can cope with old, black, gay, disabled people remains an open question. So too does its links with middle range theorising and mainstream sociological theory. Such questions indicate that our work in developing and expanding the sociology of disability is only just beginning.

There is one final issue that needs to be discussed and that concerns the distinction I make between participatory, applied and action research (alternative 1) and emancipatory research (alternative 2). To return to the game metaphor I used earlier, it seems to me that the former approaches are concerned to allow previously excluded groups to be included in the game as it is whereas emancipatory strategies are concerned about both conceptualising and creating a different game, where no one is excluded in the first place.

From a slightly different perspective Morrow makes a similar point:

The debates about postmodernism have brought to the fore all of the accumulated issues suppressed by the positivist vision of restoring order through science following the collapse of the religious worldview. Given the waning of this totalising modernist vision, we are confronted with its dialectical opposite: infinite fragmentation, difference and particularity as ineluctable features of social life and the foundational limits of social inquiry.

(Morrow & Brown 1994:320)

However, he goes on to make the point that

The perspective of critical theory involves an attempt to mediate between totalising unification and anarchic fragmentation. The central claim of such a balancing act is that it is our historical understanding of social determination that allows us to envisage alternative worlds.

(Morrow & Brown 1994:320)

These alternative worlds are what Abberley (1995), elsewhere in this volume, calls Utopias, and elsewhere in this chapter I refer to as a different game.

Zarb (1992), however, has argued that the distinction between participatory and emancipatory research is a false one in that the latter will only be achieved when the material as well as the social relations of research production are overthrown: in other words when disablist late-capitalism or post-modernity have been replaced by a different kind of society. Until then, participatory research is all we have got unless we want to return to positivist or interpretive approaches.

I can live with that as long as participatory research is seen as part of the journey to Utopia: for me this is a society where people with impairments live and flourish alongside everyone else but where disabling barriers and disablist values and attitudes have disappeared. My problem with much postmodernist emancipatory research (e.g. Lather 1991) is that there is no Utopia. The challenge to existing structures of power is all; it becomes the end in itself and not the means to something better.

Conclusions

This chapter has attempted to provide a brief history of the sociology of disability. Additionally, it has suggested that confronting the hegemony of disability as it is currently produced within the old sociological paradigm is no simple task and requires us to audit our own work as well as the work of others. Such an audit involves a re-evaluation of our ontological, epistemological and methodological assumptions about disability. Finally, and central to this re-evaluation, we can only comprehend, challenge and change the hegemony that is disability by understanding the interrelations between these ontological, epistemological and methodological levels.

In this chapter I have attempted to do this in respect of my own work as well as the work of other sociologists working in the area of disability. Whether the framework I have used to do it is of any use is a question I cannot answer. About one thing I am clear; if we do make full use of the extraordinarily rich theorising about disability that has gone on in recent years, then sociology will be enriched as a discipline and disabled people may be provided with the theoretical tools to emancipate themselves.

Acknowledgements

I am grateful to all the participants who took part in the seminar in Hull in October 1994 and, in particular, to Colin Barnes and Len Barton for their specific contributions to the development of this chapter.

References

Abberley, P. (1987) 'The concept of oppression and the development of a social theory of disability' *Disability, Handicap & Society,* Vol. 2, No. 1, pp. 5–19.

Abberley, P. (1995) 'Work, Utopia and impairment' Chapter 4, this volume.

Ainley, S., Becker, G. & Coleman, L. (Eds) (1986) *The Dilemma of Difference: A Multidisciplinary View of Stigma.* London: Plenum Press.

Albrecht, G. (1976) *The Sociology of Physical Disability and Rehabilitation.* Pittsburgh: University of Pittsburgh Press.

Albrecht, G. (1992) *The Disability Business*. London: Sage.

Barnes, C. (1990) *The Cabbage Syndrome: The Social Construction of Dependence*. Lewes: Falmer.

Barnes, C. (1991) *Disabled People in Britain and Discrimination*. London: Hurst & Co.

Barnes, C. (1996) 'Theories of disability and the origins of the oppression of disabled people in Western Society' Chapter 3, this volume.

Becker, H. (1963) *Outsiders*. New York: Free Press.

Bourne, J. (1980) 'Cheerleaders and ombudsmen: a sociology of race relations in Britain' *Race & Class*, Vol. XXI, No. 4, pp. 331–52.

Bury, M. B. (1982) 'Chronic illness as biological disruption' *Sociology of Health and Illness*, No. 4 pp. 167–87.

Bury, M. B. (1991) 'The sociology of chronic illness: A review of research and prospects' *Sociology of Health and Illness*, Vol. 13, No. 4, pp. 451–68.

Bury, M. B. (1992) 'Medical, sociology and chronic illness: a comment on the panel discussion, *Medical Sociology News*, Vol. 18, No. 1, pp. 29–33.

Campling, J. (1981) *Images of Ourselves*. London: Routledge & Kegan Paul.

Darke, P. (1994) 'The Elephant Man: An analysis from a disabled perspective' *Disability, Handicap & Society*, Vol. 9, No. 3, pp. 327–42.

Davis, F. (1964) 'Deviance disavowal and the visibly handicapped' in Becker, H. (Ed.) *The Other Side*. New York: Free Press.

Davis, K. (1986) 'Pressed to death' *Coalition News*, Vol. 1, No. 4.

Davis, K. (1986) *Developing our own Definitions – Draft for Discussion*. London: British Council of Organisations of Disabled People.

Deegan, M. & Brooks, N. (Eds) (1985) *Women and Disability: The Double Handicap*. New Brunswick: Transaction Books.

De Jong, G. (1979) 'Independent living: from social movement to analytic paradigm' *Archives of Physical Medicine and Rehabilitation*, Vol. 60, pp. 435–46.

Featherstone, M., Hepworth, M. & Turner, B. (Eds.) (1991) *The Body: Social Process and Cultural Theory*. London: Sage.

Finkelstein, V. (1980) *Attitudes and Disabled People: Issues for Discussion*. New York: World Rehabilitation Fund.

Foucault, M. (1977) *Discipline and Punish: The Birth of the Prison*. London: Allen Lane.

Frank, A. (1991) 'For a sociology of the body: an analytical review' in Featherstone *et al.* (1991).

Giddens, A. (1986) (2nd Ed) *Sociology. A Brief Critical Introduction*. Basingstoke: Macmillan.

Giddens, A. (1989) *Sociology*. Cambridge: Polity Press.

Giddens, A. (1991) *Modernity and Self-Identity: Self and Society in the Late Modern Age*. Cambridge: Polity Press.

Gillespie-Sells, K. (1994) 'Getting things right' *Community Care Inside*, 31 March.

Goffman, E. (1963) *Stigma: Notes on the Management of a Spoiled Identity*. Harmondsworth: Penguin.

Gordon, G. (1966) *Role Theory and Illness: A Sociological Perspective*. New Haven: Connecticut College and University Press.

Groce, N. (1985) *Everyone Here Spoke Sign Language: Hereditary Deafness on Martha's Vineyard*. London: Harvard University Press.

Gouldner, A. (1971) *The Coming Crisis in Western Sociology*. London: Heinemann.

Gouldner, A. (1975) *For Sociology: Renewal and Critique in Sociology Today*. Harmondsworth: Pelican Books.

Haber, L. & Smith, R. (1971) 'Human deviance; normative adaptation and role behaviour' *American Sociological Review*, 36, pp. 87–97.

Hahn, H. (1988) 'The politics of physical differences: disability and discrimination' *Journal of Social Issues*, Vol. 44, No. 1, pp. 39–47.

Hammersley, M. (1992) 'On feminist methodology' *Sociology*, Vol. 26, No. 2, pp. 187–206.

Hevey, D. (1992) *The Creatures That Time Forgot: Photography and Disability Imagery*. London: Routledge.

Hill, M. (1994) 'Gettings things right' *Community Care Inside*, 31 March.

Humphreys, S. & Gordon, P. (1992) *Out of Sight: The Experience of Disability 1900–1950*. Plymouth: Northcote House Publishers.

Hunt, P. (1966) (Ed.) *Stigma*. London: Chapman.

Kuhn, T. (1961) *The Structure of Scientific Revolutions*. Chicago: University Press.

Lather, P. (1991) *Getting Smart: Feminist Research and Pedagogy With/In the Postmodern*. London: Routledge.

Lemert, E. (1962) *Human Deviance: Social Problems and Social Control*. Englewood Cliffs, New Jersey: Prentice-Hall.

Marx, K. (1913) *A Contribution to the Critique of Political Economy*. Chicago.

Merton, R. (1968) *Social Theory and Social Structure*. New York: Free Press.

Morris, J. (1989) *Able Lives: Women's Experience of Paralysis*. London: Women's Press.

Morris, J. (1991) *Pride against Prejudice*. London: Women's Press.

Morris, J. (1992) 'Personal and political: a feminist perspective in researching physical disability,' *Disability, Handicap & Society*, Vol. 7, No. 2, pp. 157–166.

Morrison, E. & Finkelstein, V. 'Broken arts and cultural repair: the role of culture in the empowerment of disabled people' in Swain *et al.* (1993).

Morrow, R. with Brown, D. (1994) *Critical Theory and Methodology*. London: Sage.

Oliver, M. (1983) *Social Work with Disabled People*. Basingstoke: Macmillan.

Oliver, M. (1986) 'Social policy and disability: some theoretical issues' *Disability, Handicap & Society*, Vol. 1, No. 1, pp. 5–18.

Oliver, M. (1990) *The Politics of Disablement*. Basingstoke: Macmillan, and New York: St Martins Press.

Oliver, M. (1992) 'Changing the social relations of research production' *Disability, Handicap & Society*, Vol. 7, No. 2, pp. 101–15.

Oliver, M., Zarb, G., Silver, J., Moore, M. & Salisbury, V. (1988) *Walking into Darkness: The Experience of Spinal Injury*. Basingstoke: Macmillan.

Parsons, T. (1951) *The Social System*. New York: Free Press.

Reason, P. (Ed.) (1988) *Human Inquiry in Action: Developments in New Paradigm Research*. London: Sage.

Robinson, I. (1988) *Multiple Sclerosis*. London: Routledge.

Rowan, J. (1981) A dialectical paradigm for research, in Reason, P. & Rowan, J. (Eds) *Human Inquiry: A Source Book of New Paradigm Research*. Chichester: John Wiley & Son.

Ryan, J. & Thomas, F. (1980) *The Politics of Mental Handicap*. Harmondsworth: Penguin.

Safilios-Rothschild, C. (1970) *The Sociology and Social Psychology of Disability and Rehabilitation*. New York: Random House.

Scambler, G. (1989) *Epilepsy*. London: Routledge.

Scott, R. (1970) *The Making of Blind Men*. London: Sage.

Shakespeare, T. (1993) *Disability, Handicap & Society*, Vol. 8, No. 3, pp. 249–64.

Shakespeare, T. (1994a) 'Cultural representations of disabled people: dustbins for disavowal' *Disability and Society*, Vol. 9, No. 3, pp. 283–300.

Shakespeare, T. (1994b) 'Conceptualising disability: impairment in sociological perspective' PhD Thesis, University of Cambridge.

Sieglar, M. & Osmond, M. (1974) *Models of Madness: Models of Medicine*. London: Collier Macmillan.

Silver, R. & Wortman, C. (1980) 'Coping with undesirable life events' in Gerber, J. and Seligman, M. (Eds.) *Learned Helplessness, Theory and Applications*. London: Academic Press.

Stuart, O. (1992) 'Race and disability: what type of double disadvantage' *Disability, Handicap & Society*, Vol. 7, No. 2, pp. 177–88.

Sutherland, A. T. (1981) *Disabled We Stand*. London: Souvenir Press.

Swain, J., Finkelstein, V., French, S. & Oliver, M. (Eds.) *Disabling Barriers and Enabling Environments*. London: Sage Publications in Association with the Open University.

Twaddle, A. (1969) 'Health decisions and sick role variations' *Journal of Health and Social Behaviour*, 10, pp. 195–215.

UPIAS (1976) 'Fundamental principles of disability' London: Union of the Physically Impaired Against Segregation.

Walker, A. & Townsend, P. (1981) (Eds) *Disability in Britain: A Manifesto of Rights*. London: Martin Robertson.

Zarb, G. (1992) 'On the road to Damascus: first steps towards changing the relations of research production' *Disability, Handicap & Society*, Vol. 7, No. 2, pp. 125–38.

Zola, I. (1979) 'Helping one another: a speculative history of the self-help movement' *Archives of Physical Medicine and Rehabilitation*, Vol. 60.

CHAPTER 3

Theories of disability and the origins of the oppression of disabled people in western society

COLIN BARNES

Since the politicisation of disability by the international disabled peoples movement (Davis, 1993; Driedger, 1989; Oliver, 1990) a growing number of academics, many of whom are disabled people themselves, have reconceptualised disability as a complex and sophisticated form of social oppression (Oliver 1986) or institutional discrimination on a par with sexism, heterosexism and racism (Barnes 1991). Thus, theoretical analysis has shifted from individuals and their impairments to disabling environments and hostile social attitudes (Barnes 1991; Barton 1989; Finkelstein 1980; Oliver 1983; Oliver and Barnes 1991). It is argued, however, that these studies have, to a greater or lesser degree, undervalued the role of culture, which here refers to a communally held set of values and beliefs (Douglas 1966), in the oppression of disabled people (Shakespeare 1994).

This chapter will explore the relationship between culture and the oppression of disabled people. It is divided into three distinct but interrelated sections. The first provides a brief overview of socio-political approaches to disability. The second examines cultural variations in perceptions of impairment, and the third looks at social responses to people with impairments in western culture prior to industrialisation, with particular emphasis on developments in Britain – the birthplace of industrial capitalism (Marx 1970). It will show that disability or the oppression of disabled people can be traced back to the origins of western society, and the material and cultural forces which created the myth of 'bodily perfection' or the 'able-bodied' ideal.

Socio-political explanations of disability

In broad terms, socio-political analyses of disability can be divided into two distinct but interrelated groups; one American and the other British. Based firmly in American traditions of structural functionalism and deviance theory, the former explains the 'social construction' of the problem of disability as an inevitable outcome of the evolution of contemporary society. The latter draws heavily on the materialist theories of Marx and Engels (1970) and suggests that disability and dependence are the 'social creation' of a particular type of social formation; namely, industrial capitalism.

However, both these approaches tend to undervalue the impact of western culture in the oppression of disabled people. This has, however, become something of a focus for writers concerned with the experience, rather than the production, of both impairment and disability.

Functionalist accounts of the emergence of disability

With their emphasis on meaning, identity and the process of labelling, American sociologists during the 1960s explored the relationship between impairment and disability. By focusing on the process of stigmatisation and the social construction of dependence by rehabilitation professionals, writers such as Erving Goffman (1968) and Robert Scott (1970) challenged the orthodox view that the problems associated with disability were the direct outcome of individually based impairments and/or medical conditions. These insights, coupled with the radicalisation of young disabled Americans in the Movement for Independent Living (ILM) led Gerben de Jong to usher in what Mike Oliver later termed the 'social model of disability' (Oliver 1983) by proclaiming that attitudinal and environmental factors are at least as important as impairment in the assessment of disability (de Jong 1979).

Deborah A. Stone (1984) developed the argument further. She maintains that all societies function through a complex system of commodity distribution, the principle engine of which is work. But since not everyone is able, or willing, to work, a second system based on perceptions of need develops. Through a largely historical account of social policy, particularly in the nineteenth century in the USA, Britain and Germany, Stone shows how access to the needs-based system is determined by both medical and political considerations. Hence, the 'social construction of disability' is explained with reference to the accumulation of power by the medical profession and the state's need to restrict access to the state-sponsored welfare system.

A variation on this approach can be found in the work of Wolf Wolfensberger. Focusing on the recent experience of western societies, Wolfensberger argues that the social construction of disability and dependence is a latent but essential function of the unprecedented growth of 'human service industries' in the post-1945 period. Whilst all these agencies have manifest or stated purposes or functions, it is the latent or unacknowledged functions which are the most powerful. These are the unacknowledged functions of human services which are achieved in subtle and indirect ways. He maintains that in a 'post primary production economy' such as America or Britain where human service industries have become increasingly important, their unspecified function is to create and sustain large numbers of dependent and devalued people in order to secure employment for others. This is in marked contrast to their stated function which is to rehabilitate such people back into the community (Wolfensberger 1989).

Gary L. Albrecht (1992) takes this one stage further by arguing that 'disability' is produced by 'the disability business'. This is in contrast to perceptions of disability as a medical condition, a form of social deviance, and/or a political or minority group issue. Drawing upon what limited anthropological and historical sources there are in this field (see below) he shows how the kind of society in which people live creates particular types of impairment and disability. He traces the ways in which the 'mode of production' – the economy and how it is organised – causes particular bio-physical conditions and affects social interpretations of impairment, and how, in modern America, due to the growth of the human service sector industries and the politicisation of disability by the disabled people's movement, 'disability' and 'rehabilitation' have been commodified and thus transformed into commercial enterprise.

While each of the above represents, to a greater or lesser degree, a major challenge to medical definitions of disability, they fail to examine some of the structural factors precipitating their application. Indeed, although both Wolfensberger and Albrecht concede that issues such as poverty, race, ethnicity, gender and age are significant factors in the construction and production of disability and dependence, the central values upon which western capitalism rests – individualism, competitive free enterprise, and consumerism, for example – goes unchallenged. For these writers 'disability' as a social problem is the inevitable outcome of the evolution of industrial society.

Materialist accounts of the emergence of disability

A more critical evaluation can be found in the work of British authors, many of whom are disabled people themselves. In an important and often overlooked essay on the experience of disability, for example, the disabled activist Paul Hunt (1966) argues that because people with impairments are viewed as 'unfortunate, useless, different, oppressed and sick', they pose a direct challenge to commonly held societal values.

For Hunt, people with impairments are 'unfortunate' because they are seen as unable to 'enjoy' the material and social benefits of modern society. Because of the centrality of work in western culture they are viewed as 'useless' since they are not able to contribute to the 'economic good of the community'. They are then marked out as members of a 'minority group' in a similar position to other oppressed groups such as black people or homosexuals because like them they are viewed as 'abnormal' and 'different' (Hunt 1966).

This led Hunt to the contention that disabled people encounter 'prejudice which expresses itself in discrimination and oppression' (1966:152). Besides the inhumane treatment he had witnessed in British residential institutions, Hunt draws attention to discrimination against people with impairments in the wider community; notably, in employment, in restaurants, and in marital relationships. The last aspect of disabled people's 'challenge' to 'able-bodied' values is that they are 'sick, suffering, diseased, in pain'; in short, they represent everything that the 'normal world' most fears – 'tragedy, loss, dark, and the unknown' (Hunt 1966:155). Clearly, the relationship between material considerations and cultural perceptions of disabled people is central to Hunt's understanding of the experience of impairment and disability in western society.

Almost a decade later the Union of the Physically Impaired Against Segregation (UPIAS), of which Hunt was a member, made the crucial distinction between impairment and disability. The former, in common with the traditional medical approach, relates to individually based bio-physical conditions, but the latter is about the exclusion of disabled people from 'normal' or mainstream society. Thus, disability is 'the disadvantage or restriction of activity caused by a contemporary social organisation which takes no or little account of people who have physical impairments and thus excludes them from participation in the mainstream of social activities' (UPIAS 1976:14). This definition was later broadened to accommodate all impairments – physical, sensory, and intellectual – by other organisations of disabled people such as The British Council of Organisations of Disabled People (BCODP), Britain's national umbrella for organisations controlled and run by disabled people (Barnes 1991; Oliver 1990).

Adopting a materialist approach to history, Vic Finkelstein (1980), also a member of UPIAS, argued that disability is an outcome of the development of western industrial society. He divides history into three distinct sequential phases. Phase One broadly corresponds to the feudal period in Britain immediately prior to industrialisation where economic activity consisted primarily of agrarian or cottage-based industries – a mode of production, he maintains, which does not preclude people with impairments from participation.

But in Phase Two, round about the nineteenth century, when industrialisation took hold, people with impairments were excluded from employment on the grounds that they were unable to keep pace with the new factory-based work system. As a consequence, they were segregated from the mainstream of economic and social activity into a variety of residential institutions. Finkelstein's Phase Three, which is only just beginning, will see the eventual liberation of disabled people from such oppression through the development and use of technology, and the working together of people with impairments and their helpers toward commonly held goals.

For Finkelstein, disability is a paradox which emerged in Phase Two – the development of western capitalist society. On the one hand disability implies 'a personal tragedy, passivity and dependence' (Finkelstein 1980:1). On the other, it can be seen as societal restriction and discrimination. In Phase One, people with impairments were dispersed throughout the community; but in Phase Two, because of the emergence of large-scale industry with production lines geared to 'able-bodied norms' and 'hospital based medicine' (p. 10) they were separated from their social origins into a clearly defined devalued group. Phase Three will witness the end of the paradox as disability will be recognised as social restriction only.

An aid to understanding rather than an accurate historical statement, Finkelstein's analysis has been criticised for being simplistic and overoptimistic. It is simplistic in that it assumes a simple relationship between the mode of production and perceptions and experiences of disability (see below). It is too optimistic in its assumption that technological development and professional involvement will integrate disabled people back into society. Technology for disabled people can be disempowering as well as empowering and, hitherto, professional vested interests have proved one of the biggest barriers to disabled people's empowerment (Barnes 1990; Oliver 1986; 1990).

A more comprehensive discussion of the transition to capitalism and its implications for disabled people is provided by Mike Oliver in *The Politics of Disablement* (1990). Drawing on each of the above Oliver provides a materialist account of the creation of disability which places 'ideology' – a set of values and beliefs underpinning social practices – or culture at the centre of the analysis. Consequently, economic development, the changing nature of ideas, and the need to maintain order during industrialisation influenced social responses to, and therefore the experience of, impairment. The rise of the institution as a mechanism of both social provision and social control, and the individualisation and medicalisation of 'social problems' under capitalism precipitated the emergence of the individualistic medical approach to disability. For Oliver the 'personal tragedy theory' of disability has subsequently achieved 'ideological hegemony' (Gramsci 1971) in that it has become naturalised, taken for granted and almost all-embracing.

Unlike the American theorists discussed earlier, these British accounts clearly suggest that the basis of disabled people's oppression is the material and ideological or cultural changes which accompanied the emergence of capitalist society.

The experience of impairment and disability, and the role of culture

Echoing many of the concerns expressed by Paul Hunt almost three decades earlier, a number of writers working from within a predominantly feminist perspective have criticised the materialist approaches of Finkelstein and Oliver for their neglect of the individual experiences of disabled people – particularly with reference to gender (Morris 1991), minority ethnic status (Stuart 1993; Begum 1994) and impairment (Crow 1992; French 1993; 1994). This has precipitated the disabled writer Tom Shakespeare to argue that the 'social model' of disability needs to be reconceptualised to include the experience of impairment. This might be achieved, he maintains, by a more rigorous analysis of the role of culture in the oppression of disabled people.

Shakespeare contends that people with impairments are not simply disabled by material discrimination but also by prejudice. Not simply interpersonal, this prejudice is implicit in cultural representation, in language and in socialisation. Drawing on the work of feminist writers such as Simone de Beauvoir (1976) he explains this prejudice with reference to the objectification of disabled people as 'other' or to visible evidence of the limitations of the body.

He suggests that the history of disability can best be understood with reference to the work of cultural anthropologists such as Mary Douglas. Responding to deep-rooted psychological fears of the unknown, Douglas suggests, 'primitive' societies react to anomalies such as impairment by reducing ambiguity, physically controlling it, avoiding it, labelling it dangerous, or adopting it as ritual (Douglas 1966). Shakespeare argues that historical experiences such as the court jester, the freak show, the asylum and the Nazi death camps can be viewed in one or other of these categories (Shakespeare 1994).

Further, adopting a similar position to that of Susan Griffin (1984), who explains women's and black people's oppression in terms of their relationship to the body, instinct and sensuality, Shakespeare extends the analysis to include disabled people, gay men and lesbians. Thus, it is not 'disability' that non-disabled people fear but impairment as 'disabled people remind non-disabled people of their own mortality'. Thus, they are a threat – either, as Douglas (1966) suggests, to order, or, to the self-perception of western humans who view themselves as 'perfectible, all knowing . . . over and above all human beings'. He concludes by suggesting that this 'ethic of invincibility' is linked directly to notions of masculinity and potency (Shakespeare 1994:298).

In terms of advancing our understanding of the role of culture in the oppression of disabled people, particularly with respect to the experience of impairment, Shakespeare's analysis may be seen as a step forward. He rightly suggests that the cultural roots of disabled people's oppression in western society predates the emergence of capitalism. However, the main difficulty with his analysis is that by endorsing Douglas' essentially phenomenological approach, he implies that all cultures respond to impairment in essentially negative terms. In other words, prejudice against people with impairments is, in one way or another, inevitable and universal.

There are at least two problems with this perspective. First, as we shall see later, there is ample anthropological evidence that all societies do not respond to impairment in exactly the same way (Albrecht 1992; Oliver 1990; Safilios-Rothschild 1970). Second, it reduces explanations for cultural phenomena such as perceptions of physical, sensory and intellectual difference to the level of thought processes, thus detracting attention away from economic and social considerations (Abberley 1988).

The next section, therefore, will focus on cultural variations in perceptions of impairment. This is followed by a materialist explanation of the oppression of people with impairments which focuses upon the cultural antecedents of western capitalism prior to industrialisation.

Cultural variations in perceptions of impairment

The existence of impairment is as old as the human body and the earliest known societies: it is a 'human constant' (Albrecht 1992:36). From at least the Neanderthal period onward, archeologists have documented the regular appearance of individuals who would today be regarded as disabled people. Two examples are the skeleton of an elderly Neanderthal man found in Shanidar Cave

– he had an advanced state of arthritis, an amputated arm, and a head injury – and the remains of a man with severe arthritis at Chapel aux Saints. Moreover, whilst we have no idea of the prevalence of impairment in early societies – some conditions such as sensory and/or intellectual impairments, for example, would not be visible in skeletal remains – there is substantial evidence from North America, Europe, Egypt, China and Peru covering thousands of years of history showing that the incidence of impairment was common among our ancestors (Albrecht 1992).

Although anthropologists have focused primarily on culture there have been relatively few attempts to explain societal responses to people with impairments (Oliver 1990). One of the earliest and, indeed, one of the most influential, is the 'surplus population thesis'. An inevitable development of late nineteenth-century thinking – notably, liberal utilitarianism and social Darwinism (see below) – it argues that in societies where economic survival is precarious any weak or dependent individuals will be disposed of. Hence, children with impairments are killed, adults with acquired impairments are forced out of the community, and elderly people are left to die. In a study of Eskimo society conducted at the turn of the century, for example, Rasmussen (1908) gives an example of an Eskimo man and his wife severely injured in an explosion; unable to fend for themselves the woman is left to die whilst the man commits suicide.

The problem with this analysis is that there are many examples of communities where economic survival is extremely hazardous yet people with impairments remain valued members of the community. Two examples are the Dalegura, a group of Australian Aborigines (Davis 1989), and the Palute, a tribe of native Americans (Hanks and Hanks 1980). In both societies infanticide was prohibited, age was considered a sign of authority and respect, and individuals with impairments were not abandoned. Indeed, it has been recorded that the Dalegura took turns carrying a woman throughout her lifetime because she had never been able to walk. She was 65 years old when she died (Davis 1989:vii).

A second implicit theoretical explanation stems from the work of Evans-Pritchard (1937). Associated with societies dominated by strong religious beliefs, this suggests that impairments are viewed as either divine punishment or the outcome of witchcraft. For the Wapogoro, for example, epilepsy is perceived as possession by evil spirits (Aall-Jillek 1965). Apart from the fact that such explanations present religious beliefs as autonomous and the only determining factor (Oliver 1990) they tend to overshadow other studies which show that people with impairments are viewed as gifted or touched by God; hence, their status is enhanced rather than diminished (Safilios-Rothschild 1970; Shearer 1981).

A third approach is rooted in the work of Douglas (1966), discussed earlier, and Turner (1967), and rests on the notion of 'liminality'. This concept was used to explain the position of people with impairments in all societies by disabled anthropologist Robert Murphy. For Murphy, disabled people lived in a state of social suspension, neither 'sick' nor 'well', 'dead' nor 'alive', 'out of society nor wholly in it . . . they exist in partial isolation from society as undefined, ambiguous people' (Murphy 1987:112). As we have seen, societal responses to impairment are not always negative. Moreover, as with Douglas' perspective, it is an explanation firmly rooted in metaphysics which ignores social and material considerations.

The latter is particularly surprising given that in 1948 (republished in 1980) Hanks and Hanks, in a much overlooked anthropological review, had shown that cultural responses to people with impairments in non-western societies were highly variable and determined by a wide range of factors. In sociological terms these responses can be divided into two distinct but interrelated categories; namely, the mode of production and the central value system. The former includes the type of economy, the need for and the type of labour, the amount of surplus it generates, and the way it is distributed. The latter relates to the social structure – whether hierarchical or egalitarian, how achievement is defined, perceptions of age and sex, its relations with neighbouring societies, its aesthetic values 'and many more functionally related factors' (Hanks and Hanks 1980:13).

It is clear then that social responses to impairment cannot be explained simply with reference to single factors such as the economy, belief systems, or cultural relativism. They are culturally produced through the complex interaction between 'the mode of production and the central values of the society concerned' (Oliver 1990:34). Within sociology, debates about which is the primary determining factor have raged since at least Marx and Weber; for Marx and Engels (1970) it is the economy which generates a particular kind of culture or ideology and for Weber (1948) it is the converse.

The next section will focus on the history of social responses to people with impairments in western society with particular emphasis on the British experience.

Disability in western culture before industrialisation

There is evidence of a consistent bias against people with impairments in western society prior to the emergence of capitalism. Examples can be found in Greek culture, Judaeo-Christian religions and European drama and art since well before the renaissance (Barnes 1991; 1992; Shearer 1981; Thomas 1982).

It is widely acknowledged that the foundations of western 'civilisation' were laid by the ancient Greeks. Their achievements in philosophy, in the arts and in architecture have had a profound effect on the culture of the entire western world. It is often overlooked, however, that the Greek economy was built on slavery and an overtly hierarchical and violent society. Although the Greeks were renowned for asserting citizenship rights and the dignity of the individual, these were never extended to women or to non-Greeks. Moreover, they were a violent race prone to war. Greek society was made up of a collection of semi-autonomous city states constantly at war with each other – to some extent this was inevitable in order to maintain a constant supply of slaves. In addition, ever pessimistic over the fate of the soul after death, Greeks asserted the importance of enjoyment of the pleasures of the physical world (Cahn 1990; Russell 1981).

Inevitably in this type of society physical and intellectual fitness was essential; there was little room for people with any form of flaw or imperfection. Indeed, the Greek obsession with bodily perfection found expression in infanticide for children with impairments and in competitive sports. In Sparta, one of the two most important Greek city states, when children were born they were inspected by the city elders; if they were deemed in any way 'weakly', they were exposed to the elements and left to die (Tooley 1983). Greek males were expected to compete both individually and collectively in the pursuit of physical and intellectual excellence.

These preoccupations were reflected in Greek philosophy and culture. The Greek gods and goddesses were the model against which all were encouraged to strive. It is significant that there was only one physically flawed God, Hephaestes, the son of Zeus and Hera. Indeed, Zeus practised a sort of infanticide by banishing his son from heaven. Later Aphrodite, the goddess of love, takes pity on Hephaestes and marries him. Yet the marriage did not last as she takes an able-bodied lover, Ares, because her husband is a 'cripple'. The now familiar association between impairment, exclusion and impotency is clear.

Moreover, the link between impairment as a punishment for sin also has its roots in Greek culture. For example, Sophocles' famous tale of Oedipus Rex who, after discovering he has committed incest by marrying his mother, blinds himself as retribution.

Additionally, Greek architecture has, throughout history, exerted a considerable influence over building design in Europe and America (Riseboro 1979). As a consequence, a great many public buildings present major access difficulties for people with mobility-related impairments (Davenport 1995).

However, when the Romans conquered Greece they absorbed its cultural legacy and passed it on to the rest of the known world as their empire expanded. Roman society was a slave-based economy, espoused individual citizenship rights, was highly militaristic, and had both materialistic and hedonistic values. Like the Greeks, the Romans were enthusiastic advocates of infanticide for 'sickly' or 'weak' children, often drowning them in the river Tiber in Rome. Those whose impairments were not visible at birth were treated harshly. For example, in the infamous Roman games 'dwarfs' were made to fight women for the amusement of the Roman people (Readers Digest 1986:116). Consider, too, the verbal abuse encountered by the Emperor Claudius prior to his ascendancy to the imperial throne following Caligula's assassination from both the Roman nobility and Roman Guards because of his multiple impairments (Graves 1934).

Nevertheless, both the Greeks and Romans developed 'scientifically' based treatments for people with acquired impairments. Aristotle, for example, attempted to study deafness and Galen and Hypocrites tried to cure epilepsy which they saw as a physiological rather than a metaphysical problem (Thomas 1982). The Romans developed elaborate hydrotherapy and fitness therapies for acquired conditions. But such treatments were only generally available to the rich and powerful (Albrecht 1992).

Some of these features are also manifest in Judaeo-Christian religious traditions – one of, if not the, principal source of contemporary western morals and values. Influenced by Greek society since the time of Alexander the Great (Douglas 1966) the Jewish culture of the ancient world perceived impairments as ungodly and as the consequence of wrongdoing. Indeed, much of Leviticus is devoted to a catalogue of human imperfections which preclude the possessor from approaching or participating in any form of religious ritual (Leviticus, 21:16–20). But unlike other major religions of the period, the Jewish faith prohibited infanticide. This became a key feature of subsequent derivatives, Christianity and Islam, as did the custom of 'caring' for the 'sick' and the 'less fortunate' either through alms giving or the provision of 'direct care' (Davis 1989).

The opposition to infanticide and the institutionalisation of charity is probably related to the fact that Jewish society was not particularly wealthy. It was predominantly a pastoral economy dependent upon the rearing of herds of cattle, goats and sheep, as well as on commercial trade (Albrecht 1992). In addition, unlike their neighbours, the Jewish people were a relatively peaceful race, prone to oppression themselves rather than the oppression of others. In such a society people with impairments would almost certainly have been able to make some kind of contribution to the economy and the wellbeing of the community. Furthermore, in its infancy Christianity was a religion of the underprivileged, 'slaves and women' (Readers Digest 1986:118) charity, therefore, was fundamental to its appeal and, indeed, its survival.

Following the fall of Rome in the fifth century AD, western Europe was engulfed by turmoil, conflict and pillage. Throughout the 'Dark Ages' the British Isles comprised a myriad of everchanging kingdoms and allegiances in which the only unifying force was the Christian Church. Given the violent character of this period it is likely that social responses to people with impairments were equally harsh.

But by the 13th century, and in contrast to much of the rest of Europe, a degree of stability had been established in the British Isles. Furthermore, there is substantial documentary evidence that in England, a separate kingdom since the tenth century, all the prerequisites of a capitalist economy, without factories, were already firmly in place. These included a developed market economy, a geographically mobile labour force, and the commodification of land. 'Full private ownership had been established (and) rational accounting and the profit motive were widespread' (Macfarlane 1979:196).

Further, an indication of English society's attitude to dependence, and by implication impairment, is evident in the property transfer agreements of the period. When surrendering property rights to their children, elderly parents were often forced to ask for very specific rights in return. For 'it is clear that without legal protection in a written document they could have been ejected from the property which was no longer their own' (Macfarlane 1979:141). Until the 17th century, people rejected by their families and without resources relied exclusively on the haphazard and often ineffectual tradition of Christian charity for subsistence. People with 'severe' impairments were usually admitted to one of the very small medieval hospitals in which were gathered 'the poor, the sick and the bedridden'. The ethos of these establishments was ecclesiastical rather than medical (Scull 1984).

However, during the 16th century the wealth and power of the English Church was greatly reduced because of a series of unsuccessful political confrontations with the Crown. There was also a steady growth in the numbers of people dependent on charity. This was the result of a growing population following depletion due to plagues, successive poor harvests, and an influx of immigrants from Ireland and Wales (Stone 1984). Hence, the fear of 'bands of sturdy beggars' prompted local magistrates to demand an appropriate response from the central authority; the Crown (Trevelyan 1948). To secure their allegiance, the Tudor monarchs made economic provision for those hitherto dependent upon the Church. The Poor Law of 1601, therefore, is the first official recognition of the need for state intervention in the lives of people with impairments. But a general suspicion of people dependent on charity had already been established by the statute of 1388 which mandated local officials to discriminate between the 'deserving' and the 'undeserving' poor (Stone 1984).

Moreover, although 'English individualism' was well entrenched by the 13th century, the Church remained a formidable force in English and European culture. Besides offering forgiveness and a democratic afterlife in a frequently hostile world where for many life could be 'nasty, brutish and short' (Hobbes 1983) the Christian Church asserted and retained its authority by propagating and perpetuating fear of the Devil and of diabolical influence. The biblical link between impairment, impurity and sin was central to this process. Indeed, St Augustine, the man credited with bringing Christianity to mainland Britain at the end of the sixth century, claimed that impairment was 'a punishment for the fall of Adam and other sins' (Ryan and Thomas 1987:87).

People with impairments provided living proof of Satan's existence and of his power over humans. Thus, visibly impaired children were seen as 'changelings' – the Devil's substitutes for human children. The *Malleus Maleficarum* of 1487 declared that such children were the product of the mothers' involvement with sorcery and witchcraft (Haffter 1968). The religious leader and scholar accredited with the formation of the Protestant reformation Martin Luther (1485–1546) proclaimed he saw the Devil in a disabled child; he recommended killing them (Shearer 1981). Moreover, Luther was the author of one-third of all books published in Germany between 1517, when he argued the heresy, and 1522. In the following 20 years, 430 editions of his biblical and theological translations came out and were distributed throughout European society. Moreover, 'Protestant literature spoke directly to the new middle class which read no Latin and which was the agent of the new capitalism' (Inglis 1990:15).

Perhaps unsurprisingly, these beliefs are also reflected in medieval literature and art. Probably the most famous example is Shakespeare's Richard the Third, written in the late 16th century. Although the real King Richard had no physical impairments (Reiser 1992) Shakespeare portrays him as twisted in both body and mind. Since he cannot succeed as a lover because of his deformity he is determined to succeed as a villain. People with impairments were also primary targets for amusement and ridicule during the middle ages. Keith Thomas' (1977) analysis of the joke books of Tudor and Stuart England illustrates beautifully the extent of this dimension of the oppression encountered by disabled people at that time. Besides references to the other so-called timeless universals of 'popular' humour such as foreigners, women, and the clergy, every impairment 'from idiocy to insanity to diabetes and bad breath was a welcome source of amusement' (Thomas 1977:80–1). Additionally, visits to Bedlam were a common form of amusement for the socially well placed, and the practice of keeping 'idiots' as objects of entertainment was prevalent among the aristocracy (Ryan and Thomas 1987).

The 18th century witnessed a significant intensification of the commercialisation of land and agriculture, and the beginnings of industrialisation. It also heralded in the 'Age of Reason' (Russell 1948) with its emphasis on 'scientific rationality' and social progress, and the emergence of liberal utilitarianism – a philosophy of secular individual and rational self interest (Abercrombie, Hill and Turner 1984) which, in political terms, legitimates policies favouring the majority at the expense of the few. Taken together these developments provided a new-found legitimacy for already well-established myths and practices from earlier times. Thus, the 19th century is synonymous with the emergence of disability in its present form. This includes the individualisation and medicalisation of the body (Armstrong 1983), the systematic exclusion of people with impairments from the mainstream of community life (Scull 1984) and, with the emergence of Social Darwinism and the Eugenics Movement, 'scientific' reification of the age-old myth that, in one way or another, people with any form of physical and or intellectual imperfections pose a serious threat to western society (Jones 1986; Kevles 1985).

Today, the importance and desirability of bodily perfection is endemic to western culture. In terms of the oppression of disabled people, it finds expression in genetic engineering, pre-natal screening, selective abortion, and the withholding and/or rationing of medical treatments to children and adults with impairments (Morris 1991; Shearer 1981; Rogers 1994), institutional discrimination against disabled people in education, employment, welfare systems, the built environment and the leisure industry (Barnes 1991), and the proliferation of 'able-bodied' values and the misrepresentation of disabled people in all forms of the communications media (Barnes, 1992; Gartner and Joe 1987; Hevey 1992). Moreover, it is only within the last decade or so that this cultural or ideological hegemony has begun to be seriously challenged.

Conclusion

This chapter has examined the origins of disability in western society. It has shown that while social responses to impairment are by no means universal there has been a consistent cultural bias against people with impairments throughout recorded history, and that this phenomenon has been ignored, undervalued, or misinterpreted by the principal socio-political theorists working in this field. Although functionalist approaches have presented something of a challenge to traditional medical explanations of disability, they have failed to acknowledge the disabling tendencies of western culture. In contrast, materialist analyses have argued that the basis of disabled people's oppression is founded upon the material and cultural changes which accompanied the emergence of western capitalism in the 19th century. Others, working from a largely feminist/phenomenological perspective, have suggested that the oppression of disabled people can only be understood with reference to both metaphysical and structural forces, and that this is reflected in both the interpersonal relations between people with and without impairments, and within western culture since before capitalism.

It is evident that the cultural oppression of people with impairments can be traced back to the very foundations of western society. At its core lies the myth of bodily and intellectual perfection or the 'able-bodied' ideal. Although historically this construct has been interpreted in a variety of ways and finds expression in several different forms, there can be little doubt that it exercises a considerable influence on the lived experience of disabled people as well as on other oppressed groups such as women, for example. It is clear, however, that this phenomenon can be explained with reference to material and cultural forces rather than to metaphysical considerations and assumptions. Thus, prejudice, in whatever form it takes, is not an inevitable consequence of the human condition, it is the product of a particular form of social development associated with western capitalism. If we wish to eliminate prejudice, therefore, we must arrest and transform that development. In addition to economic and political initiatives this must include the construction of a culture which acknowledges, accommodates and celebrates human difference, whatever its cause, rather than oppresses it.

By placing the myth of the 'body perfect' and the interaction between the material and cultural forces which sustain it at the centre of future sociological accounts of disability, and, indeed, of other forms of societal oppression, sociologists can make a considerable contribution to this process.

Acknowledgements

Some of the material contained in this paper is based on current research on Measuring Disablement in Society funded by the Economic and Social Research Council. (Award no. R000235360)

58   *Theoretical Developments*

References

Aall-Jillek, L. (1965) 'Epilepsy in the Wapogoro tribe' Acta Psychiat, *Scand* No. 61, pp. 57–86.

Abercrombie, N., Hill, S. and Turner, B. S. (1984) *The Penguin Dictionary of Sociology*. London: Penguin.

Abberley, P. (1988) 'The body silent: a review' *Disability, Handicap & Society*, Vol. 3, No. 3, pp. 305–7.

Albrecht, G. L. (1976) *The Sociology of Physical Disability and Rehabilitation*. Pittsburgh: The University of Pittsburgh Press.

Armstrong, D. (1983) *The Political Anatomy of the Body*. Cambridge: Cambridge University Press.

Barnes, C. (1990) *Cabbage Syndrome: The Social Construction of Dependence*. Lewes: Falmer.

Barnes, C. (1991) *Disabled People in Britain and Discrimination: A Case for Anti-Discrimination Legislation*. London: Hurst and Co.

Barnes, C. (1992) *Disabling Imagery and the Media: An Exploration of Media Representations of Disabled People*. Belper: The British Council of Organisations of Disabled People.

Barton, L. (Ed.) (1989) *Disability and Dependence*. Lewes: Falmer.

Begum, N. *et al.* (Eds.) (1994) *Reflections*. London: Central Council for the Education and Training of Social Workers.

Cahn, M. (Ed.) (1990) *Classics of Western Philosophy: 3rd Edition*. Indianapolis: Cambridge.

Crow, L. (1992) 'Renewing the social model of disability' *Coalition*, July, pp. 5–9.

Davenport, J. (1995) 'Part M, access and disabled people', a seminar paper presented in the Disability Research Unit in the School of Sociology and Social Policy, University of Leeds, 10 February.

Davis, A. (1989) *From Where I Sit: Living With Disability in an Able Bodied World*. London: Triangle.

Davis, K. (1993) 'On the movement' in Swain, J., *et al. Disabling Barriers: Enabling Environments*. London: Sage, pp. 285–93.

De Beauvoir, S. (1976) *The Second Sex*. Harmondsworth: Penguin.

De Jong, G. (1979) 'The movement for independent living: origins, ideology and implications for disability research' in Brechin, A. & Liddiard, P. (1983) *Handicap in a Social World*. Milton Keynes: Hodder and Stoughton in Association with the Open University Press, pp. 239–48.

Driedger, D. (1989) *The Last Civil Rights Movement*. London: Hurst & Co.

Douglas, M. (1966) *Purity and Danger*. London: Routledge & Kegan Paul.

Evans-Pritchard, E. (1937) *Witchcraft, Oracles and Magic Amongst the Azande*. Oxford: Clarendon Press.

Finkelstein, V. (1980) *Attitudes and Disabled People*. Geneva: World Health Organisation.

French, S. (1993) 'Disability, impairment or something in-between' in Swain, J., *et al. Disabling Barriers: Enabling Environments*. London: Sage, pp. 17–26.

French, S. (Ed.) *On Equal Terms: Working With Disabled People*. London: Butterworth Heinemann.

Gartner, A. and Joe, T. (Eds.) (1987) *Images of the Disabled. Disabling Images.* New York: Praeger.

Goffman, E. (1968) *Stigma: Notes on the Management of Spoiled Identity.* Harmondsworth: Penguin.

Graves, R. (1934) *I Claudius.* London: Penguin Books.

Gramsci, A. (1971) *Selections from the Prison Notebooks.* London: Lawrence and Wishart.

Griffin, S. (1984) *Women and Nature.* London: The Women's Press.

Haffter, C. (1968) 'The changeling: history and psychodynamics of attitudes to handicapped children in european folklore' *Journal of the History of Behavioural Studies*, No. 4.

Hanks, J. and Hanks, L. (1980) 'The physically handicapped in certain non-occidental societies' in Philips, W. and Rosenberg, J. (Eds.) *Social Scientists and the Physically Handicapped.* London: Arno Press.

Hevey, D. (1992) *The Creatures Time Forgot.* London: Routledge.

Hobbes, T. (1983) 'Leviathan' in Held, D. (Ed.) *States and Societies.* Oxford: Martin Robertson, pp. 68–71.

Inglis, F. (1990) *Media Theory: An Introduction.* London: Basil Blackwell.

Jones, G. (1986) *Social Hygiene in the Twentieth Century.* London: Croom Helm.

Kevles, D. J. (1985) *In the Name of Eugenics.* New York: Alfred A. Knopf.

Macfarlane, I. (1979) *The Origins of English Individualism.* Oxford: Basil Blackwell.

Marx, K. (1970) *Capital Vol. 1.* London: Lawrence and Wishart.

Marx, K. and Engels, F. (1970) *The German Ideology: Students Edition.* London: Lawrence and Wishart.

Morris, J. (1991) *Pride Against Prejudice.* London: The Women's Press.

Murphy, R. (1987) *The Body Silent.* New York: Henry Holt.

Oliver, M. (1983) *Social Work with Disabled People.* London: Macmillan.

Oliver, M. (1986) 'Social policy and disability: some theoretical issues' *Disability, Handicap & Society*, Vol. 1, No. 1, pp. 5–19.

Oliver, M. (1990) *The Politics of Disablement.* London: Macmillan.

Oliver, M. and Barnes, C. (1991) 'Discrimination, disability and welfare: from needs to rights' in Bynoe, I., Oliver, M. and Barnes, C. *Equal Rights and Disabled People: The Case for a New Law.* London: Institute of Public Policy Research.

Rasmussen, K. (1908) *People of the Frozen North.* Philadelphia: Lippincott.

Readers' Digest (1986) *The Last Two Million Years.* London: Readers' Digest.

Rieser, R. (1992) 'Stereotypes of disabled people' in Rieser, R. and Mason, M. *Disability Equality in the Classroom: A Human Rights Issue.* London: Disability Equality in Education, pp. 98–104.

Risebero, B. (1979) *The Story of Western Architecture.* London: Herbert.

Rogers, L. (1995) 'Downs babies miss out on heart surgery' *The Sunday Times*, 24 October, p. 1.

Russell, B. (1981) *History of Western Philosophy*. London: Unwin Paperbacks.

Ryan, J. and Thomas, F. (1987) *The Politics of Mental Handicap* (Revised Edition). London: Free Association Books.

Safilios-Rothschild, C. (1970) *The Sociology and Social Psychology of Disability and Rehabilitation*. New York: Random House.

Scott, R. A. (1969) *The Making of Blind Men*. London: Sage.

Scull, A. (1984) *Decarceration (2nd edn.)*. London: Polity Press.

Shakespeare, T. (1994) 'Cultural representations of disabled people: dustbins for disavowal' *Disability & Society*, No. 9, Vol. 3, pp. 283–301.

Stone, D. A. (1984) *The Disabled State*. Macmillan: London.

Stuart, O. (1993) 'Double oppression: an appropriate starting point' in Swain, J. *et al. Disabling Barriers: Enabling Environments*. London: Sage, pp. 93–101.

Thomas, D. (1982) *The Experience of Handicap*. London: Methuen.

Thomas, K. (1977) 'The place of laughter in Tudor and Stuart England' *Times Literary Supplement*, 21 January, pp. 77–81.

Tooley, M. (1983) *Abortion and Infanticide*. New York: Oxford University Press.

Trevelyan, G. A. (1948) *English Social History*. London: Longmans Green.

Turner, V. (1967) *The Forest of Symbols: Aspects of Ndembu Ritual*. New York: Cornell University Press.

Weber, M. (1948) *From Max Weber: Essays in Sociology*, Edited with an Introduction by H. H. Gerth and C. Wright Mills, London, Routledge & Kegan Paul.

Wolfensberger, W. (1989) 'Human service policies: the rhetoric versus the reality' in Barton, L. (Ed.) *Disability and Dependence*. Lewes: Falmer, pp. 23–42.

CHAPTER 4

Work, Utopia and impairment

PAUL ABBERLEY

In this chapter I try to relate some core features of mainstream social theory to issues in the sociology of disablement. In disability theory there is a reluctance, explicable in political terms, to discuss impairment. However, it is necessary to do so if we are to develop a deeper analysis of the relationship between impairment and disability. Impairment is not 'natural' but an historically changing category; equally, not all restrictions on human activity are oppression. The sociological critique of the oppression of disabled people, which is a reflection of the 'real movement', has been effective in the last few years.

Sociological practice is related to social theory, not just in terms of concepts, tools and explanatory structures, but also of ultimate aims. The way in which a particular analysis criticises the real world is predicated upon a notion of how things could be, a Utopia. Classical social theories give participation in production a crucial importance in social integration; in their Utopias work is a need, as a source of identity. Such theories imply the progressive abolition of impairment as restrictive on the development of people's full human capacities. But as the total achievement of this aim is impossible, some non-oppressive disadvantage still remains for impaired people in such Utopias.

Feminist theory charges that such work-based theories are sexist. But much feminist research does not redefine identity separately from work, rather it expands the definition of what work is to include non-disabled women. However, some feminist research contains elements, an analysis of the body, a scepticism concerning technology, which are both materialist and critical; this may help us towards theorising a social role for impaired people in Utopia. Equally, research into social movements and on the theorisation of human needs contains elements which may be of use.

The most fundamental issue in the sociology of disability is a conceptual one. The traditional approach, often referred to as the medical model, locates the source of disability in the individual's deficiency and her or his personal incapacities. In contrast to this, the social model sees disability as resulting from society's failure to adapt to the needs of impaired people.

The World Health Organisation, for example, operates in terms of a four part medically based classification, developed by Wood (1981) known as the International Classification of Impairment, Disability and Handicap (ICIDH). This functions to link together the experiences of an individual in a logic which attributes disadvantage to nature. A *complaint*, like a spinal injury, causes an *impairment*, like an inability to control one's legs, which *disables* by leading to an inability to walk, and *handicaps* by giving the individual problems in travelling, getting and retaining a job et cetera. Thus the complaint is ultimately responsible for the handicap. A social model of disability, on the other hand, focuses on the fact that so-called 'normal' human activities are structured by the general social and economic environment, which is constructed by and in the interests of non-impaired people. 'Disability' is then defined as a form of oppression:

> the disadvantage or restriction of activity caused by a contemporary social organisation which takes no or little account of people who have physical impairments and thus excludes them from the mainstream of social activities

> (UPIAS 1976:3–4)

> The term 'disability' represents a complex system of social restrictions imposed on people with impairments by a highly discriminatory society. To be a disabled person in modern Britain means to be discriminated against

> (Barnes 1991:1)

Such a model is advanced by the Disabled Peoples International, of which the British Council of Disabled People is a member, and increasingly utilised in the field of disability studies. For a social model, both the notion of normality in performance and the disadvantage experienced by the 'deficient' performer are oppressive social products. Thus the meaning attached to 'disability' here spans the area covered by the two WHO terms 'disability' and 'handicap'. It is such a definition, with its bipartite distinction between impairment and disability, that I employ and discuss in this paper.

Several writers (Morris 1991, 1992; Shakespeare 1993, 1994) have raised, from within the general perspective of a social model of disablement, the issue of impairment, and commented on the way in which debate on this topic tends to be frowned upon and foreclosed within the disability movement. In particular, Sally French writes:

> While I agree with the basic tenets of (the social model of disability) and consider it to be the most important way forward for disabled people, I believe that some of the most profound problems experienced by people with certain impairments are difficult, if not impossible, to solve by social manipulation (1993:17).

[But] when discussing these issues with disabled people who adhere strictly to the definition of disability as 'socially imposed restriction' I am either politely reminded that I am talking about 'impairment' not 'disability', or that the problems I describe have nothing to do with lack of sight but do indeed lie 'out there' in the physical and social environment; my lack of perception of this is put down to my prolonged socialisation as a disabled person. Being told that my definitions are wrong, that I have not quite grasped what disability is, tends to close the discussion prematurely.

(1993:19)

There are clear short-term, tactical reasons why this closure of debate occurs. In a world where impaired people are disadvantaged, discriminated against and despised it is to be expected that part of the resistance to this should initially involve a concentration on the unjust social process of disablement, and a corresponding disregard for impairment. Additionally, an analysis and a political practice which draw so heavily upon the models of anti-sexism and anti-racism are likely to reproduce with the rejection of biological explanations of social inequality a disinclination towards any discussion of physical difference. But for the fuller development of social theories of disablement, it is necessary to specify the differences, as well as the similarities, between disablement and other forms of oppression, and to work out a way of incorporating the material reality of impairment into social theories of disablement. I wish to argue that we must talk more about impairment at the level of *theory* if we are to make sense of disability, since impairment is the material substratum upon which the oppressive social structures of disablement are erected. Furthermore that impairment cannot be reduced to 'mere' difference. Thus:

A theory of disability as oppression must offer what is essentially a social theory of impairment.

(Abberley 1987:9)

To do so involves the recognition that impairment cannot be understood as an abstract category, since it always and only occurs in a particular social and historical context which determines its nature. One consequence of this is that at the point where a given impairment may be prevented, eradicated or its effects significantly ameliorated it can no longer be regarded as a simple natural phenomenon even if it were at one time correct to do so. Rather, it takes on a social aspect. Thus the experience of simple cataracts, or erosion of the hip joint, whilst once perhaps reasonably viewed as a product of nature, cannot today be seen in this country separately from the social phenomena of damaging social practices, NHS waiting lists, fund-holding queue jumping, age- and impairment-based discrimination and so on.

The withholding of treatment when it is possible and desired must be seen as a form of oppression. But what was once the substratum of impairment also slides into the superstructure of disablement, and thus of oppression, in another way. This second way is when the technical possibility of 'cure' comes to be experienced as a moral imperative by the impaired person and her family, because a social system organised around the taken-for-granted desirability of independence, work and physical normality cannot admit of exceptions to this world-view. It is assumed that impairment, if avoidable, is not to be tolerated. Thus the possibility of 'cure' leads to the ideological oppression of those who do not wish themselves, or their children, to be 'rectified'. Whilst this aspect is more difficult for non-disabled people to grasp, as indeed it is for many disabled people themselves, so socialised are we into the non-disabled view of us, it lies at the heart of the issue of the authenticity of impaired modes of being.

Such an analysis, in pointing to the falsity of the natural/social split, also indicates the necessity of a complex historical specificity to any distinction between impairment and disability. To go further:

Humans are by nature unnatural. We do not yet walk 'naturally' on our hind legs, for example: such ills as fallen arches, lower back pain and hernias testify that the body has not adapted itself completely to the upright posture. Yet this unnatural posture, forced on the unwilling body by the project of tool-using, is precisely what has made possible certain aspects of our 'nature': the hand and the brain, and the complex system of skills, language, and social arrangements which were both effects and causes of hand and brain. Man-made and physiological structures have thus come to interpenetrate so thoroughly that to call a human project contrary to human biology is naive: we are what we have made ourselves, and we must continue to make ourselves as long as we exist at all.

(Dinnerstein 1977:21–2)

In this view the notion of impairment as, in the final analysis 'natural', is not so much false, as incoherent. The 'medical model', which dissolves the social into the biological, is turned around, and impairment becomes an aspect of the social, which is defined as co-terminous with the whole history of evolved humanity. This is not to say that all restrictions on human freedom are oppressive. People are not oppressed by simple natural phenomena, such as gravitational forces. Instead, oppression results from human agency. This connection is presupposed by the fact that oppression is unjust, since questions of justice can only arise in situations where human agency is concerned. However, to recognise the inevitable historicity of impairment is not to deny its materiality. Timpanaro argues:

It is certainly true that the development of society changes men's (sic) ways of feeling pain, pleasure and other elementary psycho-physical reactions, and that there is hardly anything that is 'purely natural' left in contemporary man, that has not been enriched and remoulded by the social and cultural environment. But . . . to maintain that, since the biological is always presented to us as mediated by the 'social', the 'biological' is nothing and the 'social' is everything, would . . . be idealist sophistry.

(Timpanaro 1975:45)

To develop a theory of disability as oppression, then, involves concrete discussions of the ontological status of impairment, which is by no means exhausted by simply locating impairment within the individual and disability in society.

Functionalist sociology and disablement

In the last ten years sociology-based critiques of the existing situation of disabled people have proved analytically and politically most productive. However, this advance would not have been possible if it were only occurring in the minds of isolated individuals. Intimately involved in the genesis of these works is the real movement of disabled people in Britain, and the force of academic works resides to a large degree in the fact that they crystallise within them the beliefs, concerns and interests of the increasing number of disabled people who themselves see disablement as social process rather than personal tragedy, some of whom reject all negative evaluations of impairment. We should, however, be more precise as to which areas of sociology have been of use; it is certainly not to such an inherently conservative perspective as functionalism that disability researchers have looked for their theoretical tools. Indeed, in the hands of a sociologist like Topliss (1982), such a perspective has been identified as part of the problem. The deficiencies of such accounts stem not from individual inadequacies but from the theoretical problematic in which they operate. The thorough critique of such perspectives involves not merely the rejection of their assertions about disabled people, but the deconstruction of their notions of disability, exposing them as ideological or culturally constructed rather than as natural or a reflection of reality (Alcoff 1988).

Durkheim (1964) posits a fundamental distinction between non- or pre-industrial societies and industrial ones. In the former, social integration is characterised as based on the similarity of roles in the social division of labour, 'mechanical' solidarity. After industrialisation, with a growing separateness and distinction of the individual from the group as the division of labour is increasingly specialised and individuated, a good society is one with strong bonds of 'organic' solidarity. These bonds are constituted through the recognition of the role of others in the complex division of labour that makes up that society. The venue where this solidarity is to be forged is the occupational associations. Thus to be deprived of such a role is to be deprived of the possibility of full societal membership. Whilst some of his polemical writing, like the essay 'Individualism and the Intellectuals' (Durkheim 1971), written as an intervention in the Dreyfus Affair, places great stress upon the necessity for the good society to recognise diversity, there is no suggestion that this extends to the incorporation into society of those unable to work.

It is no accident that Topliss, operating from a functionalist perspective ultimately traceable back to the work of Durkheim, advances the following argument for the inevitability of discrimination against disabled people:

While the particular type or degree of impairment which disables a person for full participation in society may change, it is inevitable that there will always be a line, somewhat indefinite but none the less real, between the ablebodied majority and a disabled minority whose interests are given less salience in the activities of society as a whole.

Similarly the values which underpin society must be those which support the interests and activities of the majority, hence the emphasis on vigorous independence and competitive achievement, particularly in the occupational sphere, with the unfortunate spin-off that it encourages a stigmatising and negative view of the disabilities which handicap individuals in these valued aspects of life. Because of the centrality of such values in the formation of citizens of the type needed to sustain the social arrangements desired by the able-bodied majority, they will continue to be fostered by family upbringing, education and public esteem. By contrast, disablement which handicaps an individual in these areas will continue to be negatively valued, thus tending towards the imputation of general inferiority to the disabled individual, or stigmatization.

(Topliss 1982:111–2)

For Topliss the inevitable disadvantage of disabled people, in any possible society, stems from our general inability to meet standards of performance in work. This can be contrasted to other perspectives, like Interactionism, where some writers (Haber and Smith 1971) suggest that the core 'deficiency' of disabled people is an aesthetic one.

Utopias in social theory

Given the political unacceptability, for the disability movement (Bynoe, Oliver and Barnes 1991, Liberty 1994) of such perspectives, it is to the more social-critical perspectives of Marxism and feminism that writers have turned in developing their models. This has resulted in the identification and exposition of fundamental problems of disablement as socio-economic in nature. But there is also, if theories of disablement are to develop further, a need to discuss the future that the various sociological theories and perspectives we make use of hold out for impaired people. This is not for reasons of mere theoretical curiosity but because the Utopias implicit in social theories read themselves back into current analysis and consequent political theorising and practice. We need to deconstruct not just 'disability' but also the future that critical modes of analysis hold out for impaired people if we are to understand how to make use of them; we need to deconstruct Utopias. First it needs to be pointed out that such 'good societies' are envisaged and have their force as distillations of the present into real possibilities, not as mere pipedreams. In her discussion of Ernst Bloch's 'The Principle of Hope' Ruth Levitas shows how he defines Utopian thought as the Not Yet:

the expression of hope, a hope construed 'not only as emotion . . ., but more essentially as a directing act of a cognitive kind'.

(Levitas 1990:87)

She continues:

All wishful thinking . . . draws attention to the shortcomings of reality, a necessary step on the way to change. In addition the Not Yet is intended to convey not just the interdependence of want and satisfaction, but the drive from one to the other, towards change (ibid:) . . . If the assertion that Utopia is anticipatory is not to imply a wholly idealist and voluntarist view of the future, the distinction must be made between those dreams of a better life that constitute real possibilities and those that do not; Bloch is therefore driven to make a distinction between abstract and concrete Utopia. Anticipatory elements are identified with concrete Utopia . . . compensatory elements with abstract Utopia . . . the task is to reveal and recover the anticipatory essence from the dross of contingent and compensatory elements in which Utopia is dressed up in particular historical circumstances . . . For Bloch the unfinished nature of reality locates concrete Utopia as a possible future within the real; and while it may be anticipated as a subjective experience, it also has objective status.

(Levitas 1990:88–9)

Utopian thought, in this sense, would appear to be a necessary aspect of a theory of oppression in that it denotes what it would mean for that oppression to be abolished; in this sense the concept is not an evaluative one, rather it is a following through of the logic of the rejection of certain aspects of present-day society to delineate the consequences of their posited eradication. It poses the question, to any particular critical social theory, 'what are the consequences for impaired people of your good society?'

Thus whilst it is perfectly correct and necessary to explore and document the socio-economic determinants of the disablement of impaired persons, and this task must at the present time take up perhaps the vast bulk of work in the development of social theories of disablement, this is not all that needs to be done. For in order to do this effectively it seems necessary to discuss what it is that we 'anticipate' if the partial and historically conditioned demands of a section of disabled people are not to be inadvertantly elevated to general principles in the theory and politics of disablement. And for this to occur we require a consideration, from the point of view of the theory we employ to analyse the present, of impairment in a world without disablement.

Marxism and impairment

In terms of the analysis of the oppression of disabled people in capitalist societies, Marxism has provided effective tools, but in relation to Marxist Utopian thought I think we encounter profound difficulties for impaired people. Marx occasionally seems to reduce the problem of human freedom to free time, in for example the 1847 'Wage-Labour and Capital' (Marx 1969). In such a view there should be no problem for those unable to labour in Utopia: free time would occupy the whole of life. But this position is more generally ridiculed and in the 1857–8 *Grundrisse* it is asserted that 'Really free working is at the same time precisely the most damned seriousness, the most intense exertion' (Marx 1973:611). In the 1875 'Critique of the Gotha Programme' Marx makes the well-known statement that:

in a more advanced phase of communist society . . . when labour is no longer just a means of keeping alive but has itself become a vital need . . . (we may then have) from each according to his abilities, to each according to his needs.

(Marx 1974:347)

But this implies that impaired people are still deprived, by biology if not by society. Impairment, since it places a limit upon creative sensuous practice, is alienatory, for those who accept that this term should be seen as an element of a Marxist terminological canon. This is not perhaps a problem in relation to free time, since even in Utopia people would not be expected to take part in all possible recreational and cultural activities. It does, however, constitute a restriction in relation to work, which is an interaction between agent and nature which results in production of social value. Whilst the distinctions between productive, reproductive and unproductive labour are crucial to the analysis of capitalism, rather than the exploration of a Marxist

Utopia, the ability to labour in some socially recognised sense still seems a requirement of full membership of a future good society based upon Marxist theory. Whilst children as potential workers, and elderly people, as former workers, may be seen as able to assume a status in a paradise of labour, it is hard to see how, despite all efforts by a benign social structure, an admittedly small group of impaired people could achieve social integration. Following Marxist theory understood in this way, some impaired lives cannot then, in any possible society, be truly equal, since the individual is deprived of the possibility of those satisfactions and that social membership to which her humanity entitles her, and which only work can provide. For impaired people to be adequately provided for in the system of distribution, but excluded from the system of production (that is, on a superior form of welfare) would be unsatisfactory, since the impaired would still occupy the essentially peripheral relationship to society we do today. For Marxism, then, there is an identification of who you are with the work you do which transcends capitalism and socialism and enters the concrete Utopia of the future to constitute a key element of humanity, and a key need of human beings in all eras. Whilst other needs can be met for impaired people, and this can perhaps be done in a non-oppressive manner, the one need that cannot be met for those unable to labour is the need to work.

Baudrillard (1975) has referred to this basic element of Marxist thought as a romanticism of productivity. William Morris, whose *News from Nowhere* envisages a profound erosion of barriers between necessary labour and the rest of human life, therefore attributes to work a crucial role in human happiness and identity:

I believe that the ideal of the future does not point to the lessening of men's energy by the reduction of labour to a minimum, but rather to the reduction of pain in labour to a minimum . . . the true incentive to useful and happy labour is and must be pleasure in the work itself
(cited Levitas:108)

Marcuse, whilst believing that work can, in Utopia, be more pleasant than it is today, points to a deep coincidence of analysis between Marx and Freud:

Behind the Reality Principle lies the fundamental fact of scarcity . . . whatever satisfaction is possible necessitates work, more or less painful arrangements and undertakings for the procurement of the means for satisfying needs.
(Marcuse 1955:35)

Andre Gorz, at the opposite pole from Morris in his advocacy of the minimisation of socially necessary labour and the maximisation of free time, still sees purposive activity and competence as a condition of social inclusion:

the abolition of work does not mean abolition of the need for effort, the desire for activity, the pleasure of creation, the need to cooperate with others and be of some use to the community.

. . . the demand to 'work less' does not mean or imply the right to 'rest more'.

(Gorz 1982:2–3)

But this is precisely the kind of right that impaired people do demand, today and for the future.

It seems that Marxism, in any interpretation, along with allopathic medicine which has been so tied to the disablement of impaired people in the modern era, can never be other than a project of the Enlightenment. It shares with other such enterprises a Rationalist adherence to aspirations of 'perfection', and can only identify non-workers with the historically redundant bourgeoisie, one aspect of whose alienation is their failure to participate in social production. And the implications of this theoretical exploration seem remarkably similar, and equally objectionable, to those arrived at in Topliss's functionalism.

Work and disability theory

How does this feed back into analyses of disability in society today? With less than one-third of those in the relevant age-group in employment in Britain today (Martin, Meltzer and Elliot 1988), for many disabled people the demand for access to work is seen as a crucial component of the struggle for equality. This is reflected in the focus of government's feeble proposals to 'tackle' disabled peoples' oppression which focus on the workplace. Recent work (Lunt and Thornton 1994) has surveyed some of the issues involved in implementing employment policies in terms of a social model of disablement – but the aim of these policies left unexamined. At the level of more general theory, Finkelstein has pointed out repeatedly (1980, 1993):

that the predominant factor contributing to the disablement of different groups is the way in which people can participate in the creation of social wealth.

(1993:12)

He goes on to argue that since –

assumed levels of employability separate people into different levels of dependency. . . . By trying to distance themselves (groups of people with particular impairments or degrees of impairment) from groups that they perceive as more disabled than themselves they can hope to maintain their claim to economic independence and an acceptable status in the community.

(1993:14)

He cautions against doing this for what are essentially political reasons, that it will divide the movement, and points out that those who did this would be surrendering to the logic of the medical model, which they claim to reject. Now this appeal to unity and theoretical consistency, whilst appropriate to its context, seems to me to pass over an essential issue for disabled people, obscured by the romanticism of productivity – that even in a society which *did* make profound and genuine attempts to integrate impaired people into the world of work, some would still be excluded by their impairment. Whatever efforts are made to integrate impaired people into the world of work, some, in any possible work-based Utopia, will not be capable of producing goods or services of social value – 'participating in the creation of social wealth'. This is so because, in any society, certain, though varying, products are of value and others are not, regardless of the effort that goes into their production. I therefore wish to contend that just because a main mechanism of our oppression is our exclusion from social production, we should be wary of drawing the conclusion that fighting this oppression should involve our widescale inclusion in social production. As Finkelstein recognises, a society may be willing, and in certain circumstances become eager, to absorb a portion of its impaired population into the workforce, yet this can have the effect of maintaining and perhaps intensifying its exclusion of the remainder. Indeed this issue appears to be arising in a distorted form in relation to the Paralympics (BBC TV 1994), where the taking up by sponsors of aesthetically pleasing, near 'normal' sports and athletes involves the rejection of 'more disabled' participants, whose performance is seen as unpleasing and whose achievements are unvalued.

Feminist analyses

Feminism has pointed out that Marxism is deeply marked by the maleness of its originators – and never more so than in the key role assumed by work in the constitution of human social identity. It is argued that the apparent gender-neutrality of Marxist theoretical categories is in reality a gender-bias which legitimises Marxism's excessive focus on the 'masculine sphere' of commodity production. Feminist responses to this have taken a number of forms, which seem to have different implications for disabled people.

Jenny Morris argues (1991, 1992) that in so far as disabled people figure in certain feminist analyses at all it is as a burden upon women, to be eradicated in the short term through the extension of institutional care and in the long term through the eradication of impairment. She criticises feminists who produce such formulations as the following for ignoring the existence and indeed preponderence of women amongst the disabled population:

we should be mounting a much stronger criticism of present ideas of 'community care' and fighting for new forms of institutional care.

(McIntosh 1981:35)

Finch states that 'On balance it seems to me that the residential route is the only one which ultimately will offer us a way out of the impasse of caring' (1984:16). In a similar vein Dalley concludes that 'This much is certain then: the familial model of care which currently dominates is based on premises which are unacceptable to feminists' (1988:137).

The nature of the residential care advocated by such writers would, we are assured, be very different from the institutions of today, with:

a lively integrated community of individuals participating freely and fully in the social life of the group and having relationships with others outside the group, where carers and cared for collaborate.

(Dalley 1988:121)

Indeed Finch presents the whole business of depriving disabled people of their liberty as at least a precursor of Utopia –

Collective solutions (to the impasse of caring) would, after all, be very much in the spirit of a socialist policy programme. (With) a recognition that caring is labour, and in a wage economy should be paid as such . . . an additional bonus would be for the creation of additional 'real' jobs in the welfare sector.

(1984:16)

Elsewhere Morris says:

Ramazanoglu . . . justifies her failure to incorporate disabled and older women into her analysis. She writes: 'whilst these are crucial areas of oppression for many women, they take different forms in different cultures, and so are difficult to generalise about. They are also forms of difference which could be transformed by changes in consciousness' (Ramazanoglu 1989 p. 95). These are really flimsy arguments.

(Morris 1992:161)

If we follow Morris's critiques of these feminist writers we again seem drawn to the conclusion that, in terms of such theories, impaired people must remain oppressed or disappear in their Utopia. Such analyses do not redefine social membership separately from work; rather they redefine work so as to include non-disabled women amongst the ranks of potentially non-alienated workers. If that which in Marxism presents itself as a concept of human beings as genderless is in fact a conception of them as male, some feminism may equally be seen as a concept of humanity as capable of and defined by labour. Such definitions ignore, and thus perpetuate the oppression of, impaired people, the majority of whom, in Britain today at least, are women.

Feminism is, however, neither a static nor a unitary perspective, and within this diversity a number of commonly identified concerns suggest more fruitful results for the proponents of the continued existence of impaired people in a real Utopia. One aspect of this involves feminist conceptions of the human body, which are far less abstract than classical Marxist formulations. In exploring the politics of human reproductive biology, feminism opens up other aspects of our biological lives, and thus impairment, to critical reflection. Another is that it has pointed out that the traditional policy solutions for dealing with inequality – 'get a job', as well as traditional technological solutions – have not resulted in a better society for women:

One fact that is little understood . . . is that women in poverty are almost invariably productive workers, participating fully in both the paid and the unpaid work force . . . Society cannot continue persisting with the male model of a job automatically lifting a family out of poverty.

(McKee 1982:36)

In *Black Feminist Thought*, Patricia Hill Collins quotes May Madison, a participant in a study of inner-city African Americans, who has pointed out that:

One very important difference between white people and black people is that white people think you *are* your work . . . Now, a black person has more sense than that because he knows that what I am doing doesn't have anything to do with what I want to do or what I do when I am doing for myself. Now, black people think that my work is just what I have to do to get what I want.

(quoted Collins 1990:47–8)

Whilst white male non-disabled sociologists may interpret this as evidence for the thesis of the alienated or instrumental worker, we should perhaps see it as documenting the social basis of an alternative theory of social membership and identity. This negative evaluation of the significance of 'work' and 'technology' in the present is not construed as explicable in terms of 'deformations under capitalism', but is carried forward into a critique of the viability for women of a society organised around 'work' and the 'technofix'. Such issues are, I think, of significance to the development of theories of disablement. Schweickart, amongst many, represents another strand in arguing that:

The domination of women and the domination of nature serve as models for each other. Thus, science and technology have a place in a feminist Utopia only if they can be redefined apart from the logic of domination.

(1983:210)

This debate seems an important one for disability theory, both in terms of such detail as the desirability of care activities being performed by machines and of wider issues of how far it would be correct to transform impaired people to give us access to the world. Thus amongst the 'deep' issues of the relationship between human beings and nature raised within feminism are many which echo in disability theory.

Social movements and theories of need

The theoretical perspectives I have considered above seem to me to imply an important distinction between disablement and other forms of oppression. Whilst the latter involve a Utopia in which freedom can perhaps be seen as coming through full integration into the world of work, for impaired people the overcoming of disablement, whilst immensely liberative, would still leave an uneradicated residue of disadvantage in relation to power over the material world. This in turn restricts our ability to be fully integrated into the world of work in any possible society. One implication that can be drawn from this, which finds most support in classical sociological perspectives with their emphasis on the role of work in social membership, is that it would be undesirable to be an impaired person in such a society, and thus that the abolition of disablement also involves as far as possible the abolition of impairment.

The work-based model of social membership and identity is integrally linked to the prevention/cure-orientated perspective of allopathic medicine and to the specific instrumental logic of genetic engineering, abortion and euthanasia. Ultimately it involves a value judgement upon the undesirability of impaired modes of being. However, this logic allows for the integration of perhaps a substantial proportion of any existing impaired population into the social work process, but only insofar as the interface between an individual's impairment, technology and socially valued activity produced a positive outcome. Thus the abolition of an individual's disablement is ultimately dependent upon and subordinate to the logic of productivity. Recent events in China, where a 'genocidal' eugenics law has been accompanied by significant equality legislation for disabled people exemplifies this logic.

An alternative kind of Utopian theory can be seen as offering another future in so far as it rejects work as crucially definitional of social membership and is dubious about some of the progressive imperatives implicit in modern science. But such perspectives are not mere piece-meal modifications to existing ideas of Utopia. Such rejections and doubt seem also to involve a distancing from the values of 'modern' society characterised by Giddens (1990) as a system of production and control based upon industrialism, the military-industrial complex and the surveillance of social life, since such a society necessarily involves the identification of persons with what they can produce in such a system.

One mode of analysing the rejection of the instrumental rationality of the modern world is examined by Shakespeare, who explores the possibility of understanding the rise of the disability movement in terms of 'New Social Movements . . . [the] most recent fixation of sociologists' (1993:257). Whilst he considers the usefulness of a number of social movement theorists, the work of Alain Touraine is not mentioned in his discussion. This is unfortunate, since Touraine's notion of social movements places particular emphasis upon the challenge that they pose to prevailing belief systems, and takes his analysis significantly beyond the empirical.

From concrete explorations of the rise of Solidarity in Poland (1983a) and the French opposition to nuclear energy (1983b), Touraine concludes (1984) that far from being peripheral and idiosyncratic areas of study, social movements constitute a central issue for contemporary sociology. For Touraine the aim of a social movement is not simply to react against existing inequalities, but rather to working towards changing the norms and values of cultural and social life. At the same time, Touraine is at pains to assert the effects upon actors of social structure and of history. For action to produce new elements of social structure it must work through and against pre-existing institutions and cultural forms: 'A social movement is at once a social conflict and a cultural project' (1995:240). The full depth of such conflictual projects is evidenced in his recent work (1995), where social movements are linked to critiques of the instrumental rationality which dominates whilst the Enlightenment values of reason, freedom, method, universalism and progress hold sway. For the Frankfurt school, Foucault and post-modernist analyses, modernity is seen as inevitably giving rise to the very oppressions it seeks to overcome. For Touraine, however, such critiques fail to recognise the 'self-critical' and 'self-destructive' nature of modernity, that the value-based rationality embodied in the practice of social movements is capable of challenging, and defeating, the ascendency of production-based instrumental rationality.

Touraine thus attempts to reintroduce the notion of action and the social movement, the mobilisation of convictions based on moral conviction and personal issues, against prevailing sociological determinism. Certainly, the women's movement, a number of 'green' campaigns, action against various provisions of the Criminal Justice Act, and, as I write, the degree and kind of mobilisation against the live export of veal calves suggest that Touraine's analysis succeeds in locating significant features of modern social life which are not reducible to traditional production-based sociological explanations. As far as the disability movement is concerned, Jenny Morris has written:

The philosophy of the independent living movement is based on four assumptions:
   that all human life is of value;
   that anyone, whatever their impairment, is capable of exerting choices;
   that people who are disabled by society's reaction to physical, intellectual and sensory impairment and to emotional distress have the right to assert control over their lives;
   that disabled people have the right to full participation in society.
(1993:21)

Such assumptions contain clear counter-values to prevailing productionism, posing demands without obligation to 'earn' and strictures on as yet unachieved rights; they constitute a set of counter-values to prevailing social norms. As embodied in the practice of the movement, such ideas can be seen as coming to constitute a theoretical and practical alternative – in Touraine's terms, a social movement.

Whilst Touraine's emphasis upon action seems of particular relevance in the analysis of the disability movement, a renewed interest in human needs apparent in social philosophy over the last 20 years is also of relevance to the theorising of impaired identity. Winner of two prestigious awards, the Myrdal and the Deutscher prizes, Doyal and Gough's *A Theory of Human Need* (1991) surveys and evaluates work in this field and attempts to draw up an agenda for need satisfaction. Their conceptualisation of disability is overwhelmingly in terms of the medical model, and their single reference to the literature of the disability movement suggests that they have failed to grasp the issues involved, and thus to incorporate them into their general conclusions. Nevertheless, such debate is one from which disability theory can benefit and insofar as it can define itself in contradistinction to the disablist assumptions contained in such models of humanity, develop its own character.

Conclusion

It seems to me that such theoretical perspectives are fertile sources for sociological theories of disablement to draw upon in their future development. Politically, they unite the interests of all impaired people. Analytically, they provide ways of understanding the oppression of all disabled people as a socially created category, not just of that subsection, however large it may be, which may potentially become part of the world of work. This is by no means to deny that the origins of our oppression, even for those with jobs, lie in our historical exclusion, as a group, from access to work, nor is it to oppose campaigns for increasing access to employment. It does, however, point out that a thoroughgoing materialist analysis of disablement today must recognise that full integration of impaired people in social production can never constitute the future to which we as a movement aspire. If we must look elsewhere than to a paradise of labour for the concrete Utopia that informs the development of theories of our oppression, it is not on the basis of classical analyses of social labour that our thinking will be further developed. Rather it involves a break with such analyses, and an explicit recognition that the aspirations and demands of the disability movement involve the development and proselytisation of values and ideas which run profoundly counter to the dominant cultural problematic of both left and right. This is not a matter of choice, but of the future survival of alternative, impaired, modes of being.

I am thus arguing that we need to develop theoretical perspectives which express the standpoint of disabled people, whose interests are not necessarily served by the standpoints of other social groups, whether dominant or oppressed, of which disabled people are also members. Such sociology involves the empowerment of disabled people because knowledge is itself an aspect of power. Disabled people have inhabited a cultural, political and intellectual world from whose making they have been excluded and in which they have been relevant only as problems. Scientific knowledge, including sociology, has been used to reinforce and justify this exclusion. A new sociology of disablement needs to challenge this 'objectivity' and 'truth' and replace it with knowledge which arises from the position of the oppressed and seeks to understand that oppression. Such sociology requires an intimate involvement with the real historical movement of disabled people if it is to be of use. Equally, such developments have significance for the mainstream of social theory, in that they provide a testing ground for the adequacy of theoretical perspectives which claim to account for the experiences of all of a society's members.

References

Abberley, P. (1987) 'The concept of oppression and the development of a social theory of disability' *Disability, Handicap & Society*, Vol. 2, No. 1, pp. 5–19.

Alcoff, L. (1988) 'Cultural feminism versus post-structuralism: the identity crisis in feminist theory' *Signs*, Vol. 13, No. 3:405–36.

BBC TV (1994) July 11th *'Disability and Dollars'*.

Barnes, C. (1991) *Disabled People in Britain and Discrimination*. London: Hurst & Co.

Baudrillard, J. (1975) *The Mirror of Production* (trans. M. Poster). St Louis: Telos Press.

Bynoe, I., Oliver, M. and Barnes, C. (1991) *Equal Rights for Disabled People – the Case for a New Law*. London: Institute for Public Policy Research.

Collins, P. (1990) *Black Feminist Thought*. London: Harper Collins.

Dalley, G. (1988) *Ideologies of Caring – Rethinking Community and Collectivism*. London: Macmillan.

Dinnerstein. D, (1977) *The Mermaid and the Minotaur: Sexual Arrangements and Human Malaise*. New York: Colophon.

Doyal, L. and Gough, I. (1991) *A Theory of Human Need*. London: Macmillan.

Durkheim, E. (1964) *The Division of Labour in Society*. Illinois: Glencoe.

Durkheim, E. (1969) 'Individualism and the intellectuals' (trans. Lukes S. and J.), *Political Studies*, XVII, pp. 14–30.

Finch, J. (1984) 'Community care: developing non-sexist alternatives' *Critical Social Policy*, Vol. 9, No. 4, pp. 5–19.

Finkelstein, V. (1980) *Attitudes and Disabled People: Issues for Discussion*, New York: World Rehabilitation Fund.

Finkelstein, V. (1993) 'The commonality of disability' in J. Swain *et al*, (Eds) (1993) *Disabling Barriers – Enabling Environments*. London: Sage/Open University Press.

French, S. (1993) 'Disability, impairment or something in between?' in J. Swain *et al. op. cit.*

Giddens, A. (1990) *The Consequences of Modernity*. Cambridge: Polity Press.

Gorz, A. (1982) *Farewell to the Working Class – An Essay on Post-industrial Socialism*. London: Pluto Press.

Haber, L. and Smith, T. (1971) 'Disability and deviance' *American Sociological Review*, Vol. 36, pp. 82–95.

Levitas, R. (1990) *The Concept of Utopia*. Hemel Hempstead: Philip Allen.

Liberty (1994) *Access Denied – Human Rights and Disabled People*. London: National Council for Civil Liberties.

Lunt, N. and Thornton, P. (1994) 'Disability and employment: towards an understanding of discourse and policy' *Disability, Handicap & Society*, Vol. 9, No. 2, pp. 223–38.

McIntosh, M. (1979) 'The welfare state and the needs of the dependent family' in S. Burman (Ed) *Fit Work for Women*. London: Croom Helm.

McKee, A. (1982) 'The feminisation of poverty' *Graduate Woman*, Vol. 76, No. 4, pp. 34–6.

Marcuse, H. (1955) *Eros and Civilization*. New York: Vintage Books.

Martin, J., Meltzer, H. and Elliot, D. (1988) *Report 1: The Prevalence of Disability Among Adults*. London: HMSO.

Marx, K. (1969) 'Wage-labour and capital' in *Marx-Engels Selected Works* Volume 1. Moscow: Progress Publishers.

Marx, K. (1973) *Grundrisse*. Harmondsworth: Penguin Books.

Marx, K. (1974) Critique of the Gotha Programme in *The First International and After*, Political Writings Volume 3. Harmondsworth: Penguin Books.

Morris, J. (1991) *Pride Against Prejudice: Transforming Attitudes to Disability*. London: The Women's Press.

Morris, J. (1992) 'Personal and political: a feminist perspective on researching physical disability' *Disability, Handicap & Society*, Vol. 7, No. 2, pp. 157–66.

Morris, J. (1993) *Independent Lives – Community Care and Disabled People*. London: Macmillan.

Ramazanoglu, C. (1989) *Feminism and the Contradictions of Oppression*. London: Routledge.

Schweickart, P. (1983) 'What if . . . science and technology in feminist Utopias' in J. Rothschild (Ed.) (1983) *Machina ex Dea-Feminist Perspectives on Technology*. Oxford: Pergamon.

Shakespeare, T. (1993) 'Disabled people's self-organisation: a new social movement?' *Disability, Handicap & Society*, Vol. 8, No. 3, pp. 249–64.

Shakespeare, T. (1994) 'Cultural representation of disabled people: dustbins for disavowal?' *Disability and Society*, Vol. 9, No. 3, pp. 283–300.

Swain, J., Finkelstein, V., French, S. and Oliver, M. (Eds.) (1993) *Disabling Barriers, Enabling Environments*. London: Sage.

Timpanaro, S. (1975) *On Materialism*. London: New Left Books.

Topliss, E. (1982) *Social Responses to Handicap*. Harlow: Longman.

Touraine, A. *et al* (1983a) *Solidarity – An analysis of a Social Movement* (trans. D. Denby). Cambridge: Cambridge University Press.

Touraine, A. *et al.* (1983b) *Anti-nuclear Protest: the Opposition to Nuclear Energy in France* (trans. P. Fawcett). Cambridge: Cambridge University Press.

Touraine, A. (1984) 'Social movements: special area or central problem in sociological analysis?' *Thesis Eleven*, No. 9, pp. 5–15.

Touraine, A. (1995) *Critique of Modernity* (trans. D. Macey). Oxford: Basil Blackwell.

UPIAS (1976) *Fundamental Principles of Disability*. London: Union of Physically Impaired Against Segregation.

Wood, P. (1981) *International Classification of Impairments, Disabilities and Handicaps*. Geneva: World Health Organisation.

PART TWO

Disability and Education

Educational policy and provision has been the subject of particular attention from successive conservative governments. All levels of the educational system have experienced the impact of multiple changes, including the governance, funding, content and outcomes of school and post-school provision.

Through the introduction of a populace discourse concerned with questions of choice, standards and competition, previous forms of relationships and understandings with schools and LEAs have been drastically changed. Supporting these developments has been the introduction of significant legislation, including the 1981, 1988 and 1993 Education Reform Acts.

It is in this context that the chapter by Riddell seeks to examine such discourses as they are reflected in key policy documents. She argues that there is a growing tendency to reinforce an individual deficit view of special educational needs/disability and that, in the present political climate, there is a need for sociological theory based on the recognition of commonalities crossing the diverse experiences of disabled people. Future theorising needs to take account of both the material and cultural basis of oppression and endeavour to involve disabled people as active agents within the research process.

In the chapter by Slee, the analysis is focused on the development of theories of disability with a particular consideration of the potential of theory to analyse recent policy questions. He is interested in how critical sociological accounts of disability can be moved from the periphery to the centre in policy-making arenas. The arena of education provides the general policy context and specific attention is given to the management of integration policy. Slee argues that the discourse of integration does little to challenge the pervasiveness of exclusionary theories of disability within state education authorities' policies.

Considering the issue of disability and higher education, Hurst maintains that this is an important but neglected social setting in which disabled people continue to experience oppression. Using illustrations of practice from within higher educational institutions, including his own, he provides insights into both the difficulties and possibilities of implementing an inclusive policy for *all* students. He also identifies some of the difficult dilemmas that being a member of different kinds of national organisations generate for him as a researcher. While advocating the importance of theorising, Hurst highlights the continual dilemma of agreeing to modifications of the status quo within existing practice, as opposed to pursuing a more radical strategy for change.

CHAPTER 5

Theorising special educational needs in a changing political climate

SHEILA RIDDELL

Although it has been argued that there is a need for a greater focus on theory in research and writing on disability, it is worth considering why this might be regarded as a worthwhile project. First, it might be justified as a means of understanding why social institutions and relationships assume certain forms rather than others, although of course some might dismiss this type of theorising as an elite and dispensable activity. Perhaps a more important justification is that in order to challenge existing power relations, it is important to render theory explicit and offer alternative interpretations of how things are and how they might be. Abberley conveys a sense of the interactive nature of theory and action when he argues that a theory of disability:

. . . is inevitably a political perspective, in that it involves the defence and transformation, both material and ideological, of state health and welfare provision as an essential condition of transforming the lives of the vast majority of disabled people.

(1992:243)

This paper reflects the view that official policies of disability are theoretically informed and tend to offer a justification of the status quo. Written policies, however, are not simply passed down to those who implement and experience them, but are contested and possibly subverted at every stage. As Bowe and Ball noted, actors are involved in the 'processes of active interpretation and meaning-making which relate policy texts to practice' (1992:13).
In addition:

policy intentions may contain ambiguities, contradictions and omissions that provide particular opportunities for parties to the 'implementation' process, what we might term 'space' for manoeuvre.

(1992:14)

It is evidently important to pay attention not just to what is written, but also to what is enacted. In particular, the paper aims to examine critically Oliver's account of changing definitions of disability and special educational needs in the post-war period. He suggested that there had been a shift away from locating problems in the individual, through seeing them as a social construction and onto recognising them as a social creation.

(1988:28)

This chapter is in three parts. The first outlines some of the ways in which special educational needs and disability have been theorised by those with a range of interests. The second part considers the discourses reflected in a number of key policy documents and the third draws on a number of recent research accounts which provide evidence of the way in which management and market-orientated policies are threatening certain discourses and privileging others. Finally, we consider the type of theory which is likely to be helpful to disabled people in the struggle for political change. The central argument is that documents published immediately before the 1979 election victory of the Conservative Party represent a shift towards a social constructionist perspective, although internal contradictions may be evident. However, rather than there being a growing acceptance of a social creationist (or materialist) approach, as Oliver argued, the effect of recent education policies, whether market-driven or imposing tighter control from the centre, has tended to be a reinforcement of an individual deficit view of special educational needs/disability. The implications of these changes for those concerned with challenging the social and economic marginalisation of people with disabilities are considered.

Ways of theorising disability

First, let us look at a range of current theoretical perspectives, the first two of which have been reflected in official policy documents and the last three of which represent a challenge to widely accepted understandings. It should be emphasised that many accounts do not fall neatly into any of these perspectives.

Essentialist perspectives

Implicit in essentialist perspectives is the belief that a characteristic or deficit is inherent within an individual and is likely to have biological rather than social causes. A number of commentators (e.g. Jenkins 1989; Abberley 1987) have noted that scant attention has been paid to theorising disability, although some studies, whilst failing to make their theoretical position explicit, tend to reflect an essentialist perspective. For instance, epidemiological studies by Kellmer-Pringle *et al.* (1966) and Rutter *et al.* (1975) assumed that impairments were social facts which could be identified with reference to accepted understandings of normal functioning. Such studies shelved doubts about uncertain boundaries and subjective definitions in the belief that once problems were identified, appropriate medical and educational provision could be made. The view that impairments were either created or constructed by wider social forces was relatively underplayed.

Accounts of the development of special education also tended to rely upon a 'march of progress' view. For example, Thomson maintained that the growth of mental testing during the early part of the twentieth century in Scotland, used to allocate individuals to particular types of special schooling, was informed by 'the genuine desire to optimise talent and concentrate on the worth of the individual' (1983:239). An alternative interpretation suggested by Tomlinson (1982) was that, far from reflecting an enlightened concern for individual needs, the expansion of special education was driven by a desire to contain and control.

Essentialist accounts, based on the premise that problems reside within the individual independently of the social context, have often been associated with conservative political agendas. However, some accounts which employ categories of impairment may reflect a progressive agenda. Barnes (1991), for example, wished to amass evidence on the extent of discrimination against disabled people in order to promote anti-discrimination legislation. He therefore gathered official statistics, based on official categories of impairment, in relation to disabled people's experience of a number of areas including education, employment, the disability benefits system and the health and social support services. Although Barnes would undoubtedly reject an essentialist perspective, he nonetheless felt that, within the context of the struggle for anti-discrimination legislation, the extent of inequality needed to be clearly established. Official statistics, he believed, could be used to reveal the nature of structural inequality in a way which detailed individual case studies could not. It is evident, therefore, that accounts using official categories and making statistical comparisons between the experiences of different groups may be used either as a means of justifying existing inequality or as the basis for challenging such inequality. It would, therefore, be unwise to dismiss out of hand all research which might be termed positivist because of its use of statistics and official categories. Clearly, the political framework within which the research is conducted must also be taken into account.

Social constructionist perspectives

Social constructionist accounts questioned the 'reality' of impairment and suggested that, rather than residing in the individual, disability should be understood as a negative label applied by some people to others with the effect of enforcing social marginalisation. Such views represented a major challenge to the essentialist view of special educational needs, although many people are reluctant to see all impairment in terms of labelling. Barton and Tomlinson for instance, maintained that whilst there could be some agreement about the definition and boundaries of certain categories of handicap,

categories such as educationally sub-normal, maladjusted, disruptive are not normative. There are no adequate measuring instruments or agreed criteria to decide on these particular categories – for example, the inclusion of children in a category of 'disruptive' depends on value-judgements, and there can be legitimate arguments between professionals, parents etc. as to what constitutes the category.

(1986:72)

As we will see in the following section, social constructionist accounts have had a significant impact on official policy. However, they have also attracted criticism from writers such as Soder (1989), who maintained that in training programmes for teachers and social workers there was an uncritical acceptance of the symbolic interactionist theory of writers such as Goffman (1961, 1963). According to Soder, a common view in such programmes is that oppression arising from impairment has a conceptual rather than a material basis and that specialised provision, particularly in separate units, confirms negative stereotypes. In Soder's view, the anti-labelling perspective is dangerous in that it may be used to justify the destruction of specialised provision and the existence of any differences at all between disabled people and others. The argument that disability is a socially constructed category rather than having some material reality may be appealing to policy makers searching for cheap solutions. However, in Soder's view it may have negative consequences for those wishing to defend welfare provision and positive action for those with special educational needs/disability.

The two perspectives discussed thus far (the essentialist and the social constructionist) have been challenged by a number of more critical accounts which have found less favour with policy makers but have nonetheless played a significant role in challenging received understandings. These are considered in the following sections.

Materialist perspectives

Very broadly, those working within a materialist perspective maintain that the oppression of disabled people is not reducible simply to problems within the individual or within the attitudes of others, but is rooted within economic structures. As Abberley explained, the oppression of disabled people has to be accounted for in material terms, thus 'the main and consistent beneficiary must be identified as the present social order, or, more accurately, capitalism in its present historical and rational form' (1992:242) Those working within this tradition have felt the need for a more disciplined approach to the analysis of disability as oppression. Abberley, for instance asserted:

> The claim that disabled people are oppressed involves, however, arguing a number of other points. At an empirical level, it is to argue that on significant dimensions disabled people can be regarded as a group whose members are in an inferior position to other members of society because they are disabled people. It is also to argue that these disadvantages are dialectically related to an ideology or group of ideologies which justify and perpetuate this situation. Beyond this it is to make the claim that such disadvantages and their supporting ideologies are neither natural nor inevitable. Finally it involves the identification of some beneficiary of this state of affairs.
>
> (1992:253)

Whilst acknowledging that disability is always experienced within and mediated by given social and economic conditions, those adopting a materialist perspective maintain that impairments are likely to have physical causes and are not merely social constructs. An attitude of ambivalence is required, so that the forces which create disability, such as war and poverty, are opposed, but the lives of disabled people are valued. This critical stance requires the challenging of ideologies which characterise disabled people as either 'less than whole' or 'really normal'.

It should be noted that although materialist perspectives have been accepted by many activists within the disability movement, they have been criticised by others as overly reductionist because of their emphasis on the economy as the basis of disabled people's oppression. Jenkins (1991), for instance, argues that although disability is related to social class, it is also a determinant of social status in its own right. Many rights and duties of citizenship which accrue automatically to the non-disabled population, whether or not they participate in the labour market, may be granted only conditionally to disabled people. For instance, there is no guarantee that a woman identified as mentally handicapped will have the right to informed consent over medical intervention, particularly in the area of fertility. In addition, on the basis of hypothetical judgements of her ability to parent successfully, she may be denied custody of her children (Booth & Booth, 1994). Social class on its own, implying some sort of relationship to the labour market, seems unable by itself to account for the particular oppression experienced by disabled people, some of whom may never participate in waged work. The constructs of social status and social worth, in addition to social class, may be helpful in understanding the relationship of disabled people to the state in non-capitalist and in different types of capitalist societies. In particular, the disability movement needs theories which take account of changes within capitalism and variations in its manifestations as it moves, in the west at least, into a post-industrial and more disorganised form. When increasingly large sections of the population in the developed world are long-term unemployed, we need to be able to explain why and how the experiences of disabled people are different from those of the wider population.

Those adopting a Foucauldian perspective, such as Fulcher have also questioned the priority attached to class relations in determining policy outcomes. Marxist theoretical frameworks, she suggested, are 'reductionist in the sense that they use those concepts (class and capitalism) to suggest that the only significant struggle is the class struggle, or the only significant "needs" are those of capitalism.' In contrast, she suggested, '. . . struggles occur over a whole range of objectives which are significant to those engaged in them (they are not a masked manifestation of the class struggle)' (1989:16). The model she adopted in her analysis of educational policy and disability was based on a notion of discourse as theory and tactic. Thus:

In each of our social practices we seek to attain our objectives and we deploy discourse as both our theory of how that bit of the world in which we want to achieve our objective works, and as tactic, that is, as a means of attaining our objective.

(1989:15)

This way of looking at the world is optimistic in that it avoids the despair which may be induced by overly deterministic accounts, but it may be criticised for seeing inequality in local rather than global terms and paying insufficient attention to structural factors which constrain negotiation. It is evident that Foucauldian accounts have often failed to offer insight into the forces underlying power-knowledge relations. It is, for instance, not accidental that disabled people, black people and women often find themselves in positions where they lack control over hegemonic discourses. Nonetheless, as Barrett (1992) points out, one of Foucault's fundamental themes is that the quest for a founding moment which will explain everything is futile. Rather than engaging in such a quest, social investigators should attempt to identify meaning in current understandings of objects and experiences.

To summarise thus far, whilst some working within a materialist perspective conceptualised disability as arising out of economic relations in capitalist society (i.e. not purely perceptual and attitudinal), others argued for alternative mechanisms rooted in struggles over social status or competing discourses. The critique of materialist accounts has been extended by a range of writers adopting post-modernist perspectives and these are considered below.

Post-modernist perspectives

Whereas some commentators like Abberley and Oliver have argued for a more consistent theory of disability, post-modernist writers have questioned the value of such a project on the grounds that human experience is too complex and diverse to be accommodated within any single account (e.g. Maclure 1994) and all meta-narrative is oppressive (Lather 1991). Furthermore, post-modernists question whether it is possible to sustain accounts of oppression since it is impossible to establish one account of events as being superior to another and notions of emancipation are based on Enlightenment views of rationality and progress. Some feminists like Lather have argued that it is possible to retain notions of empowerment within a post-modernist paradigm. In her view empowerment means:

analysing ideas about the causes of powerlessness, recognising systematic oppressive forces and acting both individually and collectively to change the conditions of our lives . . . It is important to note that, in such a view, empowerment is a process one undertakes for oneself; it is not something done 'to' or 'for' someone.

(1991:4)

There are evident problems with such a definition of empowerment which ultimately rests on notions of the individual raising his or her awareness and challenging oppression. For instance, if there is an assumption that all accounts are equally valid and individual experience is the ultimate arbiter, then how is one to judge between competing accounts or assess the validity of claims made by other individuals or groups? If the individual, possibly allied to others, is to be responsible for his or her own empowerment, then what is to become of those who lack the economic and social power required to take this action? Lather's rejection of welfarist solutions and her individualistic notion of empowerment reads uncannily like the prescriptions of the free marketeers, whose mission during the 1980s and 1990s might be summarised as 'getting government off the backs of the people'.

A more modest application of post-modernist thinking has been proposed by Corbett. She suggested that deconstruction might be helpfully used to understand the way in which language is used as an instrument of oppression. She argued, for example, that:

Special need is no longer a helpful or positive term. It is reflective of a professional ownership, in which educational and medical definitions classify what can be special and who can claim a need. It does not relate to the new discourse of the disability movement which, like the feminist movement before it, wants to take ownership of the language which has made disabled people 'the others.'

(1993:549)

Corbett concluded her paper by maintaining that:

. . . an emergence of new and diverse perspectives on the old meanings, categories and identities can only refresh our way of seeing. We may then be able to allow special need to dissolve and to support new discourses in defining the nature of need.

(1993:552)

In her view '. . . there will be no one image which can contain special need' and there is a need for 'divergent rights of way' (p. 552) but she does not consider the possibility that the conceptualisation of disability/special educational need held by one group may be oppressive of others or that accounts may conflict with one another.

It will be interesting to see whether and how post-modernist concerns impinge on future writing and research in the area of disability/special educational needs. Such approaches may be useful in addressing the implications of multiple identities, but the rejection of theory and the emphasis on the relativity of accounts may be unhelpful to those struggling for political and social change. Nonetheless, as Acker (1994) notes in relation to feminism, responding to the challenge of post-modernism may mean that debates around social theory, as opposed to social policy, remain on the agenda. Collections like those of Barrett and Phillips (1992) and Arnot and Weiler (1993) succeed in retaining a concern with the struggle for social justice whilst recognising the complex nature of group and individual identities and questioning the adequacy of overarching theory.

Because there are strong parallels between the dilemmas facing the feminist and disability movements as they seek to come to terms with critiques of meta-narrative, it is worth considering the types of argument advanced by authors of the edited collections mentioned above. Barrett and Phillips (1992) characterised 1970s feminism as an essentially modernist movement with a high degree of similarity in the problems posed by black, radical and social feminists; all were concerned with identifying the ultimate causes of women's oppression, believing that this would provide signposts towards an agenda for change. (Liberal feminists, by way of contrast, tended to see the problem in terms of discrimination based on prejudice and irrationality, rather than some overarching first cause.) Barrett and Phillips argue that since the 1970s, as women have become increasingly aware of the complex nature of identity, there has been a gradual erosion of faith in all-embracing explanations of oppression rooted in social structures. These developments have been reflected in feminist scholarship:

Feminists have moved from grand theory to local studies, from cross-cultural analyses of patriarchy to the complex and historical inter-play of sex, race and class, from notions of female identity or the interests of women towards the instability of female identity and the active creation and recreation of women's needs and concerns.

(1992:6)

The question then arises as to whether women have anything general to say and Phillips and Barrett conclude that the political agenda of feminism still requires a collective approach:

The strategic questions that face contemporary feminism are now informed by a much richer understanding of heterogeneity and diversity; but they continue to revolve around the alliances, coalitions and commonalities that give meaning to the idea of feminism.

(p 9)

Writers in the Arnot and Weiler collection also see a future agenda in terms of a 'politics of difference', but warning notes are struck about the dangers of over-emphasising difference and relativity of meaning. Yates voiced the concern that:

. . . unpicking the silences and deconstructing the categories, disowning even the term 'woman', is a dangerous one for feminist practice. What association, what movement for change can proceed on such a basis? As well, there is the question of whether current theories produce abstractions satisfying to intellectuals, whilst losing touch with palpable discriminations and inequalities which continue to affect most women.

(1993:169)

For those involved in the disability movement, precisely the same issues arise. As we noted in the previous section, seeing the oppression of disabled people purely in economic terms ignores their diverse interests and identities. On the other hand, as I have argued elsewhere (Riddell 1993) forging political alliances has been difficult for disabled people partly because of this diversity but also because of discourses which have tended to see problems in terms of individual deficits and needs rather than within a wider social structure. Just as feminists are struggling to build a political movement whilst recognising diversity, this task would also appear to be highly important for disabled people. This is discussed more fully in the following section.

Disability movement perspectives

For those identifying with the disability movement, the central justification of theory is its ability to promote social change. Oliver (1990) describes such groups as one of a number of 'new social movements' (Touraine 1981) emerging in post-capitalist society, which despite their lack of economic power, are capable of challenging social hegemony through various means including direct action. Understanding the root causes and mechanisms of oppression based on disability is less important than engaging in political action for change and therefore an eclectic approach to theorising is adopted.

The growing power of the disability movement is visible in a number of areas including the struggle over anti-discrimination legislation. However, in emphasising the significance of new social movements there is a danger that the centrality of economic structures in reproducing inequality may be underplayed. Oliver acknowledges that:

It has to be admitted that nowhere in the world have these movements been successful in overturning the status quo. Their significance has been in placing new issues on to the political agenda, in presenting old issues in new forms and indeed, in opening up new areas and arenas of political discourse. It is their counter-hegemonic potential, not their actual achievements, that are significant in late capitalism.

(1990:130)

To summarise, it is evident that disability has been theorised in a range of different ways and that such theories have been either explicit or implicit. In all perspectives, the way in which difference is construed is crucial. Within an essentialist framework, the task of professionals is regarded to be that of identifying and thereafter providing services to meet the needs of individuals with particular categories of difficulty. Social constructionist perspectives, like versions of liberal feminism, maintain that differences are due to prejudiced perceptions which can and should be altered through rational argument. Materialist perspectives regard oppression based on disability as reflecting inequalities of social class and/or social status requiring economic and ideological change. Challenging the project of theorising altogether, post-modernists assert that the complexity of experience renders all generalisation inadequate. If notions of oppression and empowerment are to be retained at all, then these must be construed in individual terms. (It should be noted that post-modernism is beset by internal contradictions. Whilst eschewing theory, much of the work is highly theoretical). Finally, the project of disability groups operating as new social movements is not to produce absolute and unassailable theory, but to develop guiding principles to inform action for change at a particular time. As I noted at the beginning of the chapter, it is important to understand the way in which such theories have fed into official education discourses and this is my concern in the following section.

Theories of disability and official educational discourses – the Warnock legacy

As we noted earlier, Oliver argued that it was possible to discern a move in official educational discourses from essentialist through social constructionist to social creationist or materialist thinking. In this section I argue that such moves are less clear-cut and rather than there being a move towards a social creationist perspective, there has tended to be a readoption of essentialist thinking, locating difficulties within the child and drawing firm boundaries between those with special educational needs and others. Let us first, however, consider the theory informing a range of key policy documents.

The Warnock Report and post-Warnock legislation

The Warnock Report has been hailed by some (e.g. Heward & Lloyd-Smith 1990) as representing a moment of enlightenment in official thinking on special educational needs, and it is certainly possible to discern radical elements within it. The system of statutory categorisation was rejected and a notion of a continuum of needs affirmed, implying a permeable boundary between pupils with special educational needs and others. However, contradictory discourses were also evident. At the same time as arguing for a focus on the educational needs of individual children, Warnock devoted sections of the report to the problems of children with particular impairments and defended special schools on the grounds that they represented 'a highly developed technique of positive discrimination'. Warnock, it appeared, wished the balance of power to shift from a medical to an educational discourse, but was wary of moving too far in this direction. Thus, in the Report one can identify both essentialist and social constructionist paradigms.

On the position of parents, Warnock is similarly ambivalent, maintaining that they should be regarded as partners in a joint enterprise, but as noted by Kirp (1982), ultimately rejecting a rights approach. Kirp was scathing of the limited nature of the partnership offered to parents. Their subordinate status, he maintained, was even reflected in the composition of the committee which was:

. . . drawn almost entirely from the professionals who had some relation to special education . . . Its chairman, an Oxford philosophy don, was the only non-specialist. Only one of the committee's 26 members was the parent of a handicapped child. The special interest groups were unrepresented for DES affirmed it was not forming a constituent body. Despite the disproportionately high number of children who had been identified as educationally sub-normal or maladjusted, no non-white served on the committee; nor was there a lawyer who might have spoken to the relevance of a legal-rights approach; nor was there a handicapped person.

(1982:155)

Rather than moving the UK further towards a rights approach, similar to that operating within the US context, Kirp maintained that a belief in the benign discretion of professionals prevailed. In a piece of research conducted in Scotland to investigate the impact of the 1980 Act (as amended) (Riddell, Thomson and Dyer 1990), we concluded that whilst supporting the rhetoric of parental partnership, professionals were anxious to retain control over placement decisions. We decided that there was evidence to support Kirp's thesis, but also that a more critical view of the rights approach was required. Whereas Kirp maintained that such an approach in the US had released greater funding for children with special educational needs, he ignored the negative aspects of this approach, which tended to foster a climate of litigation, favour parents who were articulate and able to use the system to their advantage, and undermine the attempts of regional authorities to distribute funds in an equable manner.

The post-Warnock legislation (DES 1981; SED 1980 as amended) retains this ambivalence between social constructionist and essentialist perspectives and between rights and professional discretion approaches. Thus statutory categories of handicaps are abolished, to be replaced by a new category of children with special educational needs for whom certain bureaucratic procedures are deemed necessary. With regard to parents, provision is made for involvement at various stages of assessment and recording, but key rights of appeal are denied. To some extent, then, the Warnock Report and the accompanying legislation adopted a social constructionist view of special educational needs but competing discourses survived, reflecting an essentialist view of special educational needs and of the sovereignty of professional discretion over parents' and children's rights.

The 1978 HMI Report and guidelines on learning support

The report of Scottish HMI on provision for children with learning difficulties (SED 1978) moved closer to a social constructionist perspective than the Warnock report. The former stated explicitly that children's difficulties with reading and writing were likely to arise from unsuitable curricula and teaching methods rather than problems within the child. Placing children in segregated remedial classes to practise basic skills was seen as counter-productive, since it deprived them of the stimulation provided by the mainstream curriculum and peer group. The task of class and subject teachers was to ensure such children gained access to the curriculum through the use of differentiated teaching materials and approaches. Guidelines (SCOSDE 1990) underlined the official role of learning support staff (the term remedial teacher was no longer in use) as consultants and cooperative teachers. Individual tuition was mentioned, but given a low priority. Nonetheless, despite official acceptance of the view that the cause of learning difficulties was located in the environment rather than the child and the solution was to be tackled through the modification of the learning environment, there was evidence that both mainstream and learning support teachers found it difficult to incorporate this thinking into their practice (Allan, Brown and Munn 1991).

No document equivalent to the report of Scottish HMI was ever produced south of the Border and it is interesting to speculate on Scottish schools' apparent acceptance of social constructionist thinking in relation to provision for children with learning difficulties in mainstream schools. A possible reason for this might lie in the greater commitment to comprehensive education in Scotland (McPherson and Willms 1987), accompanied by a desire to equalise learning opportunities for all children irrespective of measured ability. Compared with the relative consensus over educational philosophy in Scotland, south of the Border there continued to be considerable ambivalence over comprehensive education in general (Reynolds & Sullivan 1987) and over the best means of tackling children's learning difficulties in mainstream schools. Clearly, however, although there may have been consensus in Scotland at national and regional level in relation to values, as Allan *et al.* indicated, uncertainty persisted at the level of the classroom.

Official discourses of special educational needs in the present policy context

Despite the mixed messages of the Warnock Report and the report of Scottish HMI on children with learning difficulties, these documents may be seen as representing a high point in the move away from essentialist views of special educational needs. It is therefore of vital importance to consider how such policies are faring within the context of present government policy, characterised by tension between different versions of conservative thinking. One policy strand seeks to impose greater control from the centre, whilst another is informed by a commitment to allowing the market to shape public services. Hartley described the tension between these imperatives thus:

At one and the same time, the discourse of education policy appears to reflect the post-modern and the modern, apparently reconciling the tension between them. The legitimatory rhetoric of ownership, choice and diversity accords with the consumerist culture of an emerging post-modernism. But the close specification of both educational targets and funding has all the hallmarks of the age of modernity.

(1994:242)

Overall, however, whether informed by an agenda of choice (e.g. parental right to choice of school, delegation of financial resources to schools) or control (the publication of outcomes on a range of performance indicators, the 5–14 programme), the policy initiatives of the present government have marked a return to a child-deficit view of special educational needs. Various aspects of these policies are now considered briefly.

Special educational needs within the 5–14 curriculum

Both the Warnock Report and the 1978 Scottish HMI Report revealed a greater acceptance of the social constructionist view of special educational needs. The 5–14 programme, introduced in the early 1990s, identified normative attainment targets and maintained that the attainment of all children should be located within this framework. Some maintain that the inclusion (if only nominally) of children with special educational needs within the 5–14 programme represents a significant breakthrough in terms of establishing their entitlement to a common curriculum. Others maintain that it restricts teachers' freedom to respond creatively to such children's needs and focuses on what they cannot do rather than on their achievements (see Weedon 1994 for further discussion of this point). Recent policy documents (SCCC 1994) have attempted to explain how the 5–14 programme may be adapted for children with special educational needs. Rather than moving further towards a social constructionist perspective, however, they have tended to support a diverse view of the origins of special educational needs, identifying social, environmental and within-child factors as potential causes. Within-child factors are given a much higher profile than in the earlier report of Scottish HMI and the term 'dyslexia', previously banished from official documents, makes a reappearance. In addition, a system of categorisation has been adopted, with sections devoted to children with physical disabilities, visual impairment, hearing impairment, moderate learning difficulties, complex learning difficulties and social, emotional and behavioural difficulties. On the basis of the most recent documents from Scottish HMI and SCCC, it would be inaccurate to say that there has been a rejection of a social constructionist approach and a return to an essentialist view of special educational needs/learning difficulties. Nonetheless, there are indications of a shift in this direction.

Financial delegation to schools

Local management of school was one of the measures introduced by the Education Reform Act and the study conducted by Lunt and Evans (1994) provides us with some preliminary insight into its effects. There are indications that, because of financial pressures, instead of investing in learning support available to any child with a learning difficulty, authorities were only likely to agree to preferential funding for individual children with a Statement of Need, thus widening the gap between these with additional resources attached and those without. Warnock's idea of the permeability of the category of special educational needs is therefore seriously undermined and the only solution for schools is to push for increasingly high levels of statementing. This shift away from general support towards individualised provision is justified by a discourse of essentialism, promoting the view that children with special educational needs are fundamentally different from others. In addition, the reduction of background levels of support in mainstream may push some parents to opt for a special school placement, where additional resources are more likely to be safeguarded.

In Scotland, although devolved school management will not be fully implemented until 1996 (1997 in special schools) there were signs that Scottish schools were likely to experience some of the same pressures as those felt by authorities south of the Border. Even before schemes were fully in place, there was evidence of an increase in rates of recording of pupils in mainstream schools. (Allan, Brown and Riddell, 1994). Although funding for children with special educational needs was to be retained centrally, many published schemes were vague on the question of how the needs of children with learning difficulties (but without a Record) were to be met. It appeared that devolved school management in Scotland was likely to underline rather than diminish the barrier between children with special educational needs and others.

The delivery of learning support in the context of 'league tables'

There is some evidence from Scottish secondary schools that the pressure for accountability of funding is challenging the model of learning support delivery promoted by the 1978 HM Report and the SCOSDE guidelines. Sally Brown, Jill Duffield and myself (Brown, Riddell and Duffield 1994) have been conducting an in-depth study of four secondary schools with the aim of identifying aspects of their culture which have particular salience for lower-achieving pupils. As a result of pressure to improve academic performance, there were moves in all schools away from mixed ability teaching in S1 and S2 in order to 'fast-track' higher-achieving pupils. Learning support, previously available to all S1 and S2 classes in certain subject areas, would be restricted to the lower sets thus reintroducing the notion that only certain types of pupil experience learning difficulty. In the two schools with more pupils of higher socio-economic status, pressure from parents of children identified as dyslexic had brought about a renewed emphasis on individual tuition in place of cooperative teaching and consultancy.

The questioning of the principle of learning support for all has been fuelled by HMI in a recent critical commentary on schools' attempts to implement the recommendations of the 1978 Report referred to earlier. In secondary schools, for instance, HMI noted (SOED 1993) that tutorial support for pupils in S1–S4 'was no more than fair in over a third of cases' (5.2, p. 14). The message appeared to be that the model of learning support based primarily on consultation and cooperative teaching had not been successful and a greater focus on individual tuition was required. Overall, within learning support provision, the swing back to a child-deficit rather than a curriculum or teacher deficit model is evident, produced, at least in part, by schools' anxiety about their performance in league tables and justified by an essentialist rather than a social constructionist discourse.

School accountability and the position of children with social, emotional and behavioural difficulties in mainstream settings

Finally, there is some evidence that definitions of 'normal' and 'deviant' behaviour are being redefined within the mainstream classroom in response to managerial pressures for school and teacher accountability. A number of writers (Fairley and Paterson forthcoming; Ball 1990) have commented on the increasing use of school effectiveness and improvement research as a means of teacher surveillance and control. Both north and south of the Border, there is an increase in the exclusion rate of pupils with social, emotional and behavioural difficulties (SEBD). Armstrong and Galloway (1994) have suggested that this is linked to the growing dominance of a managerial culture. Within such a culture, easily measurable performance indicators, including external examination results, costs and truancy are used to assess teacher and school performance. In relation to such performance indicators, pupils with SEBD are likely to have a negative effect on the school's profile since they are likely to be demanding of teacher time but achieve poorly in examinations. For these reasons, including such children in mainstream schools is likely to be regarded as imposing too great a burden and they may come to be regarded as a liability. However, Armstrong and Galloway indicate that teachers feel the need to justify the exclusion of such pupils and they may do this by redefining them as disturbed (implying a pupil deficit) rather than disruptive (implying a teacher or curriculum deficit). At the same time, teachers reconceptualise their work as teaching 'normal' children rather than those with difficulties who require 'expert' tuition. Once gatekeepers such as psychologists have accepted this definition of the situation, the way is cleared for the child to be removed.

Essentialist notions of children's difficulties, then, are being employed as a coping strategy by schools and teachers in order to justify the exclusion of pupils who are regarded as difficult to educate. The question then arises as to how this process may be resisted. There would appear to be strong arguments for comprehensive schools to use development planning, over which they have some control, to establish agendas which do not simply reflect government priorities but also wider concerns for social equity. Parents must clearly play an active part in defining such values, which need to reflect the view that schools which develop a caring approach to their pupils are likely to provide a better learning environment for all.

Parental power and special educational needs

As we noted earlier, the government has regarded parental choice as the means of ensuring competition and accountability within the education system. The implications of this policy for children with special educational needs are as yet unclear and it is possible that parents may use their power to oppose collectively practices which reproduce disadvantage. Early indications, however, do not suggest that this is what is happening. A project on policy and provision for children with specific learning difficulties in Scotland (Riddell, Brown and Duffield 1994) suggested that in this particular case parents and voluntary organisations wished to promote the view that such children represented a discrete group, whose difficulties were inherent and whose needs were quite different from the normal range of cognitive difficulties. Although opposed by the majority of educational psychologists, who tended to accept Warnock's view of a continuum of difficulties, there was evidence of some success in shifting the paradigm back towards an essentialist view. The term 'dyslexia', as opposed to specific learning difficulties, had reappeared in official government documents and a major national initiative to raise the profile of dyslexia in initial teacher education was being vigorously promoted. There were also several well-publicised cases where parents, arguing for placement in an independent special school catering for dyslexic children, mounted a successful legal challenge to the education authority's view that the child's needs could be met in the mainstream school with additional learning support (see the *TESS* 14 January 1994 which reports the case of the Kinsman family versus Tayside Region).

Far from taking on the mantle of a 'new social movement', voluntary organisations acting on behalf of dyslexic children were drawing on views of learning difficulties as individual deficits unmediated by environmental conditions. They were certainly not engaging in a radical critique of social values. However, this is certainly not to argue that *all* parents would adopt such a position. For instance, in England there have recently been a number of cases where parents have challenged the decision of the local authority to place a child in a special rather than a mainstream school. (e.g. *The Observer*, 14 November 1993, reported the case of Emma Gibbs, a sixteen-year-old with Down's Syndrome, whose parents were prosecuted by Suffolk County Council for refusing to send her to a special school. The Guardian (12 September 1994) reported Lancaster County Council's refusal to admit Nicky Crane, a boy with brain damage, to a mainstream secondary school. His parents decided to keep their child at home until the LEA agreed to their placing request and there had been public demonstrations in support of the family.) In these cases, parents were clearly challenging the education authorities' views of appropriate education, but were also raising wider questions about what is construed as 'normal' and the role of segregated schools in sustaining ideologies of essential difference.

The contrast in high-profile cases north and south of the Border is worth noting, but it should be remembered that the overall pattern of provision in England and Wales and Scotland is similar, with roughly equal proportions of children being placed in special schools. However, it may be the case that, in general, parents are pursuing individual choice more vigorously in England than in Scotland and this may lead to some parents insisting on placement in a mainstream school for their child against the advice of the professionals.

Parental views on appropriate placements for their children, and, implicitly, their understandings of special educational needs, are likely to be increasingly powerful in shaping official discourse. A Scottish study (Allan, Brown and Riddell, 1994) attempts to understand the nature of education authority policies on placement of children with special needs and how these are implemented in a climate dominated by managerial and market concerns. The report includes an analysis of national placement trends and official policy documents, interviews with local policy makers and case studies of 32 children in mainstream and special schools. Most education authority policy statements were couched in rather imprecise terms of placing children in 'the least restrictive environment' and local policy makers felt that in order to fulfil parental wishes, which might be very diverse, it was necessary to maintain both mainstream and special provision. Although it is likely that professionals still have a considerable influence over parental decisions, the weakening of education authority power means that it would be difficult for an authority to carry out a policy of total integration without the support of a strong and united parental lobby. In Scotland at the moment, it appears that the strongest pressure groups are promoting the interests of individual children or children with a particular type of difficulty rather than seeking collective solutions. Present policies may allow for collective action to promote social constructionist or materialist views of special educational needs, but there are difficulties in forging such alliances among parents who may well be contending with a range of social pressures and whose energy and resources may be severely depleted. Parents' overall preference for the mainstream or special sector in the context of their greater (but still restricted) power to choose are as yet unclear and many may find themselves in the difficult position of trying to insist that their child be treated as 'normal' and socially integrated whilst at the same time arguing for additional resourcing and, perhaps, placement in a special setting.

Conclusion

We began by considering the perspectives which may be used to conceptualise disability and special educational needs in the light of the prediction of a shift from an essentialist through a social constructionist towards a social creationist (or materialist) view. It was argued that, as well as considering the theoretical position which might be most helpful to disabled people, it was also important to examine the way in which particular policies promoted certain discourses rather than others. Whereas Warnock and the 1978 Report appeared to represent a shift away from an essentialist discourse, more recent policy documents, fuelled by attempts to increase centralised control whilst simultaneously promoting market-driven approaches, indicated a move back towards a child-deficit model and the maintenance of the boundary between 'normal' children and those with special educational needs. The emphasis on consumer power might be used by parents to critique received understandings of special educational needs and establish a collective rather than an individual approach to challenging disadvantage, but so far this did not appear generally to be the case (although of course things might change).

The question remains as to the type of theory which is most likely to be helpful to disabled children and their parents in challenging oppression and indeed whether the quest for meta-narrative should be abandoned altogether. In my view, an eclectic approach is required, borrowing from a range of theories which are likely to be helpful in understanding and challenging oppression whilst recognising that no one theory is likely to be adequate in all contexts. As Tomlinson (1985) argued, perhaps the most important question which needs to be addressed is who benefits from the dominance of particular discourses. More empirical work is needed to understand the relationship between social class, social status and disability, recognising Jenkins' argument that although there are strong links between social class and disability, social class is not by itself adequate to understand the oppression of disabled people. Foucauldian accounts are likely to prove useful in understanding local power struggles, but are probably less helpful in understanding structural constraints on action. Post-modern approaches are helpful in deconstructing official discourses and emphasising the complexity of individual experiences and understandings, but it is not easy to see how deconstruction can be used in the struggle for political change.

There are, however, dangers in theoretical eclecticism, since it is possible to sidestep the question of whether some theories are mutually exclusive. I believe that it is important to identify a theory with the greatest explanatory potential and subsequently, to explore its explanatory limits, and the point at which additional accounts are required to make sense of an existing state of affairs. In the area of disability, for instance, economically grounded theories can, to some extent, explain the position of disabled people, but an additional layer of explanation, rooted in the notion of the relative social status of disabled and able-bodied people, is required to clarify the way in which the position of disabled people differs from others who are economically marginalised. My perhaps unfashionable position, then, is that meta-narratives continue to be important, but should not be expected to explain everything and that other theoretical frameworks should be drawn upon when it becomes clear that the explanatory potential of a particular theory is exhausted.

It is perhaps unfortunate that the present growth of interest in theorising disability and special educational needs is occurring at a time when there is a wider rejection of theory and a suspicion of meta-narrative within social science. This raises the question of why we need to theorise and who should be doing the theorising.

As I stated at the start of the paper, theorising is justified both in terms of understanding why things are the way they are, but also in establishing a future agenda for social change. In the context of both the disability and the feminist movements, there is a need for a greater awareness of diversity of experience. For disabled people, this will include a closer focus on how experience differs in relation to gender, 'race,' social class and the nature of impairment. Whilst focusing on diversity, however, there is a pressing need to identify commonalities, since the recognition of shared experience is likely to form the basis of political action. This recognition of commonality is likely to form the bedrock on which theory rests and just as circumstances shift and change, theory must be reappraised. This critical stance will avoid the reification of theory and ensure that such accounts are flexible and meaningful to those whose lives they attempt to understand. In order to avoid the production of theories that are no more than hide-bound monoliths, it is important that disabled people themselves take a leading role in the area and, as Oliver (1992) has argued, there continues to be an urgent need for the democratisation of research relations. We are at last seeing some studies which include people with learning difficulties as active participants (Whittaker, Gardner and Kershaw 1990). Non-disabled researchers working in this area should bear in mind the need for humility, should listen carefully to what disabled people have to say about their work and be wary of research findings which bear the mark of academic respectability but may carry negative implications for disabled people.

Finally, although an essentialist view of special educational needs may once again be in the ascendancy in official discourse, this does not mean that all attempts to establish alternative theories and agendas for change should be abandoned. Indeed, as the new social movements have realised, a powerful reason for theorising is to challenge social hegemony. In developing alternative discourses of special educational needs, there are possibilities for alliances between teachers, pupils and parents. None of these groups is in a particularly powerful position at the moment (despite the rhetoric of consumer power) and they might decide to seek their individual salvation. There is, however, a possibility of developing understanding of the way in which historical and economic conditions interact with individual circumstances to create oppression and to use this knowledge in the struggle for social change. The government's emphasis on individualism and consumer empowerment may thus be capable of subversion, and in the future, when there is a more critical view of a market-driven approach to public service delivery, this may act as a helpful antidote to the controlling paternalism which dogged earlier welfarist approaches.

References

Abberley, P. (1992) 'The concept of oppression and the development of a social theory of disability' in Booth, T., Swann, W., Masterton, M. and Potts, P. (eds) *Policies for Diversity in Education*. London: Routledge.

Acker, S. (1994) *Gendered Education: Sociological Reflections on Women, Teaching and Feminism*. Milton Keynes: Open University Press.

Allan, J., Brown, S. and Riddell, S. (1994) *Special Educational Needs Provision in Mainstream and Special Schools: Interim Report on the Scottish Office Education Department*. Stirling: University of Stirling.

Armstrong, D. and Galloway, D. (1994) 'Special educational needs and problem behaviour: making policy in the classroom' in Riddell, S. and Brown, S. (eds) *Special Needs Policy in the 1990s: Warnock in the Market Place*. London: Routledge.

Arnot, M. and Weiler, K. (eds) (1993) *Feminism and Social Justice in Education: International Perspectives*. London: Falmer Press.

Ball, S. J. 'Management as moral technology: a Luddite analysis' in Ball, S. J. (Ed.) *Foucault and Education: Disciplines and Knowledge*. London: Routledge.

Barnes, C. (1991) *Disabled People in Britain and Discrimination Legislation*. London: Hurst & Co. in association with British Council of Organisations of Disabled People.

Barrett, M. and Phillips, A. (eds) (1992) *Destabilizing Theory: Contemporary Feminist Debates*. Oxford: Polity Press.

Barrett, M. and Phillips, A, (1992) 'Introduction' in Barrett, M. and Phillips, A. (eds) (1992) *Destabilizing Theory: Contemporary Feminist Debates*. Oxford: Polity Press.

Barton, L. and Tomlinson, S. (1984) 'The politics of integration in England' in L. Barton and S. Tomlinson (Eds.) *Special Education and Social Interests*. Beckenham: Croom Helm.

Booth, T. and Booth, W. (1994) *Parenting Under Pressure: Mothers and Fathers with Learning Difficulties*. Buckingham: Open University Press.

Bowe, R. and Ball, S. J. (1992) *Reforming Education and Changing Schools: Case Studies in Policy Sociology*. London: Routledge.

Corbett, J. (1993) 'Post-modernism and the "special needs" metaphors' *Oxford Review of Education*, 19, 4, pp. 547–53.

Department of Education and Science (1978) *Special Educational Needs (The Warnock Report)*. London: HMSO.

Fairley, J. and Paterson, L. (forthcoming) 'Scottish education and the new managerialism' *Scottish Educational Review*.

Fulcher, G. (1989) *Disabling Policies? A Comparative Approach to Education Policy and Disability*. Lewes: The Falmer Press.

Goffman, E. (1961) *Asylums: Essays on the Social Situation of Mental Patients and Other Inmates*. New York: Anchor Books.

Goffman, E. (1963) *Stigma: Notes on the Management of Spoiled Identity*. Englewood Cliffs, NJ: Prentice-Hall.

Hartley, D. (1994) 'Mixed messages in educational policy: sign of the times?' *British Journal of Educational Studies*, XXXXII, 3 230–44.

Heward, C. and Lloyd-Smith, M. (1990) 'Assessing the impact of legislation on special education policy – an historical analysis' *Journal of Education Policy* 5 (1) 21–36.

Jenkins, R. (1989) 'Dimensions of adulthood in Britain: long-term unemployment and mental handicap' in P. Spencer (Ed.) *Anthropology and the Riddle of the Sphinx: youth, maturation and ageing.* London: Routledge.

Jenkins, R. (1991) 'Disability and social stratification' *British Journal of Sociology*, 42, 4 pp. 557–76.

Kellmer-Pringle, M. *et al.* (1966) *11,000 Seven Year Olds.* London: National Children's Bureau.

Kirp, D. L. (1982) 'Professionalisation as a policy choice: British special education in comparative perspective' *World Politics*, 34 (2) 137–74.

Lather, P. (1991) *Getting Smart: Feminist Research and Pedagogy With/in the Post-modern.* New York: Routledge.

Lunt, I. and Evans, J. (1994) 'Dilemmas in special educational needs: Some effects of Local Management of Schools' in Riddell, S. and Brown, S. (eds) *Special Needs Policy in the 1990s: Warnock in the Market Place.* London: Routledge.

Maclure, M. (1994) 'Language and discourse: the embrace of uncertainty' *British Journal of Sociology of Education*, 15, 2 pp. 283–301.

McPherson, A. and Willms, J. D. (1987) 'Equalisation and improvement: some effects of comprehensive reorganisation in Scotland' *Sociology*, 21, pp. 509–39.

Oliver, M. (1988) 'The social and political context of educational policy: the case of special needs' in L. Barton (Ed.) *The Politics of Special Educational Needs.* London: The Falmer Press.

Oliver, M. (1990) *The Politics of Disablement.* London: Macmillan.

Oliver, M. (1992) 'Changing the social relations of research production?' *Disability, Handicap & Society*, 7, 2 pp. 101–14.

Reynolds, D. and Sullivan, M. (1987) *The Comprehensive Experiment.* London: Falmer.

Riddell, S., Dyer, S. and Thomson, G. O. B. (1990) 'Parents, professionals and social welfare models: the implementation of the Education (Scotland) Act 1981' *European Journal of Special Needs Education*, 5, 2, pp. 96–110.

Riddell, S. (1993) 'The politics of disability: post-school experience' *British Journal of Sociology of Education*, 14, 4, pp. 445–55.

Riddell, S., Brown, S. and Duffield, J. (1994) 'Parental power and special educational needs: the case of specific learning difficulties' *British Educational Research Journal*, pp. 327–45.

Riddell, S., Brown, S. and Duffield, J. (1994) 'The social and institutional context of effectiveness: Four case studies of Scottish schools' Paper presented to the British Educational Research Association Conference, University of Oxford, 8–11 September 1994.

Rutter, M., Cox, A., Tuplir, C., Berger, M. and Yule, W. (1975) 'Attainment and adjustm .t in two geographical areas: the prevalence of psychiatric disorder' *British Journal of Psychiatry*, 126.

SCOSDE (Scottish Committee for Staff Development in Education) (1990) *Award Bearing Courses Within the Three Tier Structure: Guidelines for Diplomas in Special Educational Needs.* Edinburgh: SCOSDE.

SCCC (Scottish Consultative Council on the Curriculum) (1993) *Support for Learning: Special Educational Needs Within the 5–14 Curriculum.* Dundee: SCCC.

Scottish Office Education Department (1993) *Standards and Quality in Scottish Schools A Report by HM Inspectors of Schools.* Edinburgh: HMSO.

SED (Scottish Education Department) (1978) *The Education of Pupils with Learning Difficulties in Primary and Secondary Schools in Scotland A Progress Report by HM Inspectors of Schools.* Edinburgh: HMSO.

Soder, M. (1989) 'Disability as a social construct: the labelling approach revisited' *European Journal of Special Needs Education,* 4, 2 pp. 117–29.

Thomson, G. O. B. (1983) 'Legislation and provision for the mentally handicapped child in Scotland' *Oxford Review of Education,* 9, 3, pp. 233–40.

Tomlinson, S. (1982) *A Sociology of Special Education.* London: Routledge.

Tomlinson, S. (1985) 'The expansion of special education' *Oxford Review of Education,* 11, 2, pp. 157–65.

Touraine, A. (1981) *The Voice and the Eye: An Analysis of Social Movements.* London: Macmillan.

Weedon, C. (1994) 'Learning difficulties and mathematics in Riddell, S. and Brown, S. (eds) *Special Educational Needs Policy for the 1990s: Warnock in the Market Place.* London: Routledge.

Whittaker, A., Gardner, S. and Kershaw, J. (1990) *Service Evaluation by People with Learning Difficulties.* London: The Kings Fund Centre.

Yates, L. (1993) 'Feminism and Australian State Policy: Some Questions for the 1990s' in Arnot, M. and Weiler, K. (eds) (1993) *Feminism and Social Justice in Education: International Perspectives.* London: Falmer Press.

CHAPTER 6

Clauses of conditionality: the 'reasonable' accommodation of language

ROGER SLEE

A fundamental challenge confronting the development of sociologies of disability concerns receptions of and responses to theory. The political elasticity of language is central. In the development and generalisation of inclusive education policy linguistic veneers are applied both to advance and to conceal competing agendas. A paradigm may be appropriated to describe quite contradictory aims and practices. Researchers such as Ball (1987; 1988; 1990a), Bowe, Ball & Gold (1992), Bash and Coulby (1989) and Power (1992) identify this process in the deployment of a discourse of 'choice' and 'local management' to deepen central control over curriculum, teaching and the organisation of schools in the wake of the British Education Reform Act.

A similar tactic is reflected in the different but unreconstructed language employed by those who have hitherto presided over special education services. Formerly a medical model of disability was advanced to mark and marginalise 'special students'. Different vocabularies, which espouse rights and equity, are now used to describe the cosmetic adjustments to traditional practices which, when applied, maintain the powerlessness of disabled students, their families and their advocates, and privileges those professionals who work 'in their best interests'. The attempt to fuse two antithetical discourses of disability is theoretically flawed.

Responding to this conceptual slippage, this chapter is concerned both with the production and employment of sociologies of disability. The first part of this discussion considers the development of social theories of disability. The second section will focus upon the implications of theories of disability for educational practices.

Social theory: redefinition and reach

Considering the way in which 'linguistic omissions' have forced women to occupy the 'dark corners' of the senior management space in Australian bureaucracy, Eleanor Ramsay identifies the centrality of the form and construction of language in the process of oppression.

> ... the absence of terms which accurately and adequately describe women's experience of certain aspects of our oppression ... contributes to the construction of women's oppression, perpetuates key processes which are integral to this oppression and simultaneously prevents any protest against these processes, even at the level of analysis and description.
>
> (Ramsay 1993:44)

Lexical adjustments fall short of fundamental changes to social theory and behaviour.

> Much feminist debate over the last two decades has been focused on the generation of non-sexist terminology and the elimination of sexist and misogynist expressions ... In response, educational and employing authorities in Australia and other English speaking countries, particularly within the public sector, have taken action such as the issuing of guides to non-sexist language use in an effort to diminish the use of sexist stereotyping and prejudices in written and spoken language ... These activities and their results have been characterised as producing an acceptable language surface but have been criticised for stopping short at that surface rather than challenging and exposing the sexist substructure beneath it.
>
> (Ramsay 1993:44)

The project requires intervention into the text to reconstruct meaning, 'to force new meanings', as opposed to patriarchal interpretations of women's narratives, which describe the world experienced from a number of sites or vantages. Ramsay's discussion of language, personal experience and oppression has its parallels in the generation of social theories of disability.

Ramsay rejects the oppressive form and meaning of patriarchal language and its attempts to find a space for the accommodation of women in the world it constructs. There is also a concern that in the generation of feminist language and theory diversity is shunned in preference to single-theory explanations which provide cohesive intellectual closure for complex social relations. Similar themes emerge when plotting the development of sociological theories of disability. Suspicion is quite properly summoned when the non-disabled produce vocabularies and theoretical models to explain disability. Moreover, 'border-crossings' (Giroux 1992) are apposite when considering the narratives of disability. Structural and post-structural accounts of the world must enter into a dialogue to provide space for the many voices of disability. In this way it is possible to delineate the 'deep structure' of disablement while also filling in the fine-grain detail of its lived experiences.

By implication, if we pursue Ramsay's theme, the non-disabled have to rethink the position they take in the development of theories of disability. The outside knowledge of 'experts' is potentially theoretically and politically offensive. This is at the heart of Len Barton's discussion [see Chapter 1] of the need for dialogue between the disabled and non-disabled in the establishment of alliances. Added to this is the diversity and particularity of 'impairments' and disabilities which ought to resonate through new theories and languages of disablement.

Responding to the absence of 'good sociology' in theorising disability, Abberley (1987) critiques the construction of meaning in the widely employed bifurcation of impairment as 'personal tragedy' and 'disability' as social responses.

The latter position, at least in its more worked out forms, presents handicap as totally the product of social meanings, in other words reducible to 'attitudes'. It implies that change in attitudes could abolish disability. Claims about the social origin of impairment, however, are directed at the explication of the social origin of what are material and biological phenomena, and should be understood not as dissolving these material elements into attitudes and ideas, but rather as pointing to the inextricable and essential social elements in what constitutes a material base for ideological phenomena. Thus such a view does not deny the significance of germs, genes and trauma, but rather points out that their effects are only ever apparent in a real social and historical context, whose nature is determined by a complex interaction of material and non-material factors.

(Abberley 1987:12)

For Abberley, theorising disability necessitates a careful structural analysis of the material conditions of production and the historical specificity, as opposed to decontextualised individual pathology, of impairment. Such a theoretical perspective is liberating in its capacity to turn the gaze away from the individual towards the conditions of the world they inhabit.

Michael Oliver (1989, 1990) pursues this consideration of disability through an analysis of Western capitalist political economy. Expunging historical specificity and social context through individualising impairment invites the deployment of the medical model and reduces disability to the status of personal problems demanding 'expert' intervention and case management. The linguistic representation of disability according to this schemata has had hegemonic impact upon disabled and non-disabled people alike. Morris acknowledges this in citing Patricia Hill Collins' reflections on the obstructions erected by white masculine social structure and relations to Black feminist thought, codes of expression and empowerment:

Groups unequal in power are correspondingly unequal in their ability to make their standpoint known to themselves and others.

(cited in Morris 1992:158)

The beneficiaries of oppressive scenarios of personal tragedy theory have been the medical, para-medical, psychological, social work, and social policy communities along with sections of the academy (Abberley 1987, 1989; Oliver 1990). Locating the problem within individuals and demanding heroism to overcome their impairment [sic. dysfunctionality] in order to more closely approximate 'normalcy' bleaches out the collective responsibility of existing social structures and relations, founded upon capitalist definitions of productive labour, for oppression and disadvantage.

Theorising disability demands more than elaborations of functionalist theory – it invites us to relinquish the 'given' order, and to interrogate the normalising imperative of government (Rose 1989). Rose traces the expansion of the human 'psy' sciences as a project of governmentality (1989:5–8). Complex industrial and post-industrial societies demand more elaborate and pervasive mechanisms of surveillance and control over difference and dissent. Governmentality demands a sophisticated technology of regulation. Doctors and psychologists have been equal to the task of providing the benchmarks and the apparatus for calibrating difference and placing those who fall outside the social construction of normality (Cohen 1985; Edwards 1988; Rose 1989; de Swann 1990; Petersen 1994).

Jenny Morris's celebration of feminist theory's call for male sociology to create '. . . the space for an absent subject, and an absent experience . . .' (Smith 1987), and to reach beyond men using objectivity as a descriptor for their subjectivity (quoting Adrienne Rich in Morris 1992:159), is tempered by her acknowledgement of silences in feminist accounts:

Disability and old age are aspects of identity with which gender is very much entwined but they are identities which have been almost entirely ignored by feminists.

(Morris 1992:161)

Such silences are not properly addressed by adding disability and age to the list of excluded groups for consideration within the body of existing theory. Also challenged is the treatment of oppression within the calculus of compound equations such as 'double oppression' (Morris 1992). Calling for dialogue with 'new' voices to present new personal accounts as political (Morris 1992; Corbett 1994), Morris supports other disabled researchers (Finkelstein 1980; Oliver 1992; Barnes 1992) in directing questions to the nature, conduct and outcomes of research into disability which is emancipatory rather than alienating.

In a recent visit to our campus, Gaby Weiner described 'feminisms' as a theory in the making; 'one is never finished given its political, critical and praxis mandates' (Weiner 1993).

Grand narratives, in speaking for all, silence the particular and are thus misrepresentations for many they purport to speak for and to. Speaking generally about the experience of the disabled is as misleading as speaking about women as a universal descriptor. But caution may be advised here lest we are entrapped by the inertia of liberal [post-modern?] pluralism. Deferring to Morris (1992), Barton acknowledges the need for non-disabled researchers to be advised on their role as allies in what is essentially a political struggle (1994).

This represents the central focus for this discussion; how do we move critical sociological accounts of disability from the periphery to the centre in the various and disparate policy-making arenas? Perhaps the question is better reframed to consider strategies for change that bring policy into line rather than using policy to lead change. Questions of audience and reach are introduced, along with problems of strategy and the politics of research relationships (Troyna 1994a, 1994b). Acknowledging that policy is made at all levels (Fulcher 1989) and that it is a metaphor for a range of texts and actions in which contests over definition and choices are played out, my interest is in the inclusion of sociological accounts of disablement in more of the sites for policy making, for greater levels of struggle in disability policy making. This speaks to the political project of theory, to the struggle against dominant paradigms which reverberate within present governmental arrangements and processes.

This heuristic and incomplete discussion of theory is intended to provide a backdrop for some particular issues that I am struggling with. These struggles are located within education, but they remain ineluctably connected with the way in which we construct our theories of disability. Fulcher (1989) introduces us to the relationship between disability discourses and education policy as it is played out at various sites.

What follows is an attempt to locate policy in alternative theories and determine therefore the origins of the struggles and contradictions that emerge. Education provides our general policy context, with particular focus upon the management of integration policy. Integration refers to the movement of disabled students from segregated educational settings to the regular classroom. Caught within the bureaucratic gaze of education politics, integration has been constructed as a technical problematic of matching resources to students according to their level of impairment. It is perhaps the last of the compensatory educational drives. Medical and psychological discourses of disability predominate. The agenda is set by the special educational fraternity so that integration typically becomes a compensatory programme for a 'special' group of children. Consequently, despite the rhetoric, integration is seldom an inclusive educational provision. Authentic change which moves beyond the relocation of children from one site to another, together with traditional special educational practices, is undermined by the failure of education administrators, teachers, special education providers and teacher educators to eschew uncritical discourses of disability.

Education management, disablement and integration

After some years of struggling with education departments in Victoria, Queensland and New South Wales to develop inclusive educational programmes, I feel like an accessory after the fact, like an accomplice in exclusion. I may well attribute this apparent collusion to both the essentially 'normalising charter' of public education (Ball 1990b; Meadmore 1993), and to my own ingenuousness.

The language of integration provides little discursive challenge to state education authorities managing the politics of difference through policy struggles at all levels of educational administration and delivery (Fulcher 1989). Branson and Miller elaborate on this point:

'Disability', 'handicap', 'policy' – they fit together like pieces of a jigsaw puzzle, or, more correctly, they flow into one another, feed off each other, reinforcing each other, essential ingredients in a distinctly Western, distinctly capitalist mode of thought. The 'disabled', a marginalized group whose failures to satisfy the culturally specific, historically specific standards of physical or behavioural 'normality', display 'handicaps', inabilities to deal 'effectively', as individuals, with life in Western capitalist society, their 'handicaps' demanding, in the eyes of those for whom they are an 'other', a 'policy', an objective, clearly formulated, bureaucratically realizable, logical, coherent approach to dealing with/coping with, their 'handicaps'. The policy demands a 'programme' to transform the policy into practice through effective 'administration'. 'Segregation' was/is such a policy. 'Integration' is another version of the same, another sibling of the triad – disability, handicap, policy – a policy spawning programmes designed in terms of effective administration.

(Branson & Miller 1989:144)

For teachers and education administrators alike disability promises tyranny in the classroom, disturbs the organisational calm, stretches the boundaries of narrow academic curriculum offerings and assumes variety in approaches to teaching and learning. The 'disabled student' presents a less than docile body (Foucault 1979:138) to comply with the disciplinary framework and culture of schooling. The invention of the 'special needs student' as a meticulously calibrated scholastic identity (Ball 1990b:4) provides a framework for managing the problem of the disabled student. As Branson and Miller (1989) reflect, this may well be pursued through a policy of segregation or through integration. Both represent programmes for managing the implied threat of difference. Notwithstanding rhetorical claims of a new and socially just approach, integration is but the rearrangement of an old score (Slee 1993). More personal accounts testify to this (Rice 1993; Lyons 1993; Walsh 1993).

Mary Rice (1993), describing her experience of 'integration' as a parent, provides a further account of the bureaucratisation of integration in Victorian public schooling which demonstrates its reverberation with and amplification of traditional exclusionary special educational practices. The special educational gaze is intensified as integration locks into struggles over resources (Fulcher 1987). The raft of professionals engaged in the identification, assessment and support of those allowed into the 'mainstream' expands exponentially (Tomlinson 1982, 1993). Integration policy, in large measure, provides the administrative and surveillance technology for regulating the flow of 'difficult' students into the regular classroom.

Moreover, integration policy has become an ally to educational stasis as schools struggle, Canute-like, against history. This is best illustrated by observing developments in the management of disruptive behaviour in schools. Explaining and responding to increases in student resistance may be pursued through a number of theoretical positions (Furlong 1985, 1992; Slee 1995).

We might argue that schools have always been in the business of producing failure. This, historically, has not been seen as a problem for schools. The unskilled youth labour market and special schools provided a safety valve to eliminate potential resistance and reduce collateral damage to the status quo. Application of the label 'failure' to individual students deprob-lematised and depoliticised the issue of 'rights of passage' in schooling (Barton 1987). The disappearance of the youth labour market (Polk 1988; Polk & Tait 1990; Freeland 1992), together with the utilisation of education as an instrument of 'youth policy' and micro-economic reform (White 1990; Marginson 1993), means that schools have to live with their failures. Having no other options young people endure the pain of failure and schooling (Furlong 1992). Apart from the street, there is nowhere else to go. Schooling, for an increasing number of young people, does not promise a successful transition into the adult world of work, higher education or training.

The virtual disappearance of the unskilled labour market provides ample space for an expanding special educational industry. This can be observed in the increased expenditure on special educational needs, the expansion of professional appointments (Tomlinson 1993) to service their 'need', and the redefinition of young people in classrooms (Slee 1993).

A sociological reading of disruption has little appeal for education administrators. Its implications for fundamental changes to pedagogy, curriculum and school organisation render it too difficult to confront. Teachers, struggling to maintain control in classrooms, look longingly for the quick-fix behaviour programme offered by the likes of Glasser's 'Reality Therapy' (1965; 1986), Canter's 'Assertive Discipline' (1976), Gordon's 'Teacher Effectiveness Training' (1974) or Rogers' 'Decisive Discipline' (1989).

Far more appealing are the psychological theories of individual pathologies of emotionally or behaviourally dysfunctional children in need of therapeutic intervention. To this end Australia has been ravaged by the epidemic spread of Attention Deficit Disorder [ADD], also referred to as Attention Deficit Hyperactivity Disorder [ADHD] (American Psychiatric Association 1987; Barkley 1990; Serfontein 1990; Epstein *et al.* 1991). Diagnosis is effected by matching the behavioural symptoms of a child to an inventory of those behaviours ascribed to Attention Deficit Disorder/Attention Deficit Hyperactivity Disorder. The syndrome apparently stems from '. . . an imbalance or deficiency of one or more neurotransmitters in the brain' (Bowley & Walter 1992). Considerable diagnostic imprecision is reflected by geographical disparity in the prevalence of Attention Deficit Disorder/Attention Deficit Hyperactivity Disorder.

Attention Deficit Disorder/Attention Deficit Hyperactivity Disorder (ADD/ADHD) presents itself as a syndrome of spectacular administrative convenience. The increasing retention of young people in school devoid of post-schooling options has generated increasing conflict in schools which translates into increasing rates of suspension and exclusion (Slee 1995). The pathologising of student disruption provides a more sophisticated and pervasive technology of control than the rituals of punishment and exclusion. This diagnostic transfer is akin to what Muetzelfeldt & Bates (1992), following Habermas (1976) and Offe (1984), refer to as crisis displacement.

The complex social context of disruption in schools is reduced to an individual aetiology which can be managed through the application of a diagnostic/descriptive label, chemical interventions, withdrawal or behavioural interventions. The impairment is uncomplicated by historical or political specificity. Moreover, teacher, school culture and organisation, and curriculum are removed from the diagnostic enquiry. An increasing proportion of the integration project is directed to these not so docile bodies of disruptive or ADD/ADHD students. The 'disability' or syndrome, by invoking a medical discourse, also avoids the normative language of 'the maladjusted student'. ADD/ADHD is particularly beguiling for parents. The pathologising of the student's behaviour transforms the relationship between the child and the parent and the parent and the school. Where once they were having to account for their 'bad' child to school authorities, they now have a special needs child. Added to this is the promise of treatment and or cure. Methylphenidate [Ritalin], a central nervous system stimulant which acts on the cerebral cortex, is frequently administered to repress hyperactivity (Barkley 1990). That Govoni and Hayes (1988:778–9) have chronicled a number of adverse effects of Ritalin such as growth suppression, anorexia, nausea, blurred vision, depression, drowsiness, dizziness and cardio-vascular complications alerts us to the need for diagnostic exactitude in the face of such risk. A minimum expectation ought to be that the disabling factors of schooling be eliminated before embarking upon such a course of treatment.

Effectively, integration provides an elaborate infrastructure for the management of normality. I return to Ramsay's (1993) consideration of 'linguistic omission'. The hegemony of integration as a variation upon the theme of special education is sustained by a sheer and misleading linguistic veneer of rights and inclusion, trumpeted (perhaps hummed is more accurate) in text and in public fora. However, as Gillian Fulcher (1989) correctly observed some time ago, the growth of a corporate discourse of disability as a problem for management through policy is dominant in the conduct of integration.

In Queensland, integration was pursued through the Education Department's social justice mandate. A special educator was appointed to manage the construction of a new way of dealing with disability in education. That this resulted in tinkering and the renaming of old exclusionary practices such as an elaborate six-tiered ascertainment schedule for resource allocation (integration is almost always argued as a resources issue) is not surprising. What is surprising is that the senior policy officers for gender, race/ethnicity, and disadvantaged schooling projects were not moved to apply their sociological imagination to the Department's theorising of disability. They too have continued to draw policy advice from those who know about disabled people: academics from the Special Education and Rehabilitation Research Centres, special educators in the field, and educational psychologists. Disabled people, parents and advocates are always pushed into the status of lobbyists. We return to our earlier questions about who writes disability theory (see Barton, Chapter 1 this volume; Morris 1992; Barnes 1992) and about whose languages we employ to that end (Ramsay 1993; Morris 1992).

The clauses of conditionality prevail: 'least restrictive environment'; 'most appropriate setting'; 'reasonable accommodation'; 'in the child's best interest'. The Australian [Commonwealth] Disability Discrimination Act 1992 (No. 135 of 1992) conspires with conditionality. Exemptions from the Act are significant. The Commonwealth Department for Immigration is one such case. Implicitly people with disabilities are still seen as a cost to the public (Hastings 1993). Schools may discriminate on the basis of disability where the inclusion of a child may cause the institution 'unjustifiable hardship' (Disability Discrimination Act No. 135, 1992, **22.4**:17).

Caveats of conditionality provide ample latitude for professional interpretations which silence the disabled person. A school principal in northern New South Wales has reportedly resisted the admission of a student who uses a wheelchair. His defence is that it would compromise the safety of 'normal' students if there was an emergency evacuation and they were trapped in corridors behind the student in the wheelchair!

Whilst visiting Australia, Bonnie Tucker [Professor of Law at Arizona State University] provided an incisive comparison between Australian and American legislation (Tucker 1994). The essential difference between the effectiveness of the legislations – Disability Discrimination Act [Australia] and Americans with Disabilities Act [United States] – appertains to their origins. American legislation evolved from hard-won litigation mounted by disabled people and their advocates. Together with a more litigious culture, this has meant a greater awareness across disability groups and organisations of the legislation and its potential. This contrasts with Australia where legislation was drafted in an orchestrated governmental process and handed down. This has meant that awareness and application of the law has been limited. It would seem that the debate about disablement needs to be conducted in the widest possible fora in order to engage the polity in expunging antiquated and oppressive disability discourses as a prerequisite to comprehending and practising the spirit as well as the letter of the law.

Teachers and education administrators continue to employ the logic of exclusion to bleach out the ethical dimensions of integration. As a member of the New South Wales Department of School Education Special Needs Advisory Committee in the North Coast Region, I am constantly confronted by the plea 'for the teacher time for the other 29 children'. The arithmetic of teacher time is only applied to conspicuous disability. The 'regular kids' who demand more than their 1/30th share are seldom rebuked through this distorted view of justice. Who is the other? It is clearly not the 29 (Becker 1963). Rawls' (1972) contention that treating unequals equally does not constitute justice is salutary.

The constant paradox for this Advisory Panel is that in submissions from parents and students we are pushed in two ways. Parents of children who have been segregated in special education settings or who have had diagnostic labels applied to them plead for inclusion in the regular school and the removal of the stigmatising labels. Parents and advocates for the 'learning disabled' are equally vehement in their pleas for the attachment of labels and the recognition that this growing group of children are disabled and require special treatment. How do we respond to this?

Changing conclusions? changing discourse?

The multi-dimensional problem of theory applies. Disability continues to be uncritically accepted as uncontextualised deficient human pathology by educators. This is a significant audience pursuant to the change process. Some parents will continue to call for labels so long as educators' thinking is constrained by categorical constructions of difference and disability.

The politics of having parents and disabled people come to make their case to an Advisory Panel is a problem. The frames of reference are established and cases are mounted by parents to extract what they can from the existing order or to prove minimal disruption through their inclusion. Parents and their children are reduced to the status of beggars as they plead compensation from a benevolent authority. New languages, pursuant to the reconstruction of an inclusive school culture, will not be conceived within this context.

Barton's (1994) reflexive questions about the basis of the relationship between disabled and non-disabled researchers and activists in this project have great importance. Whose theory counts? A group of parents in central Queensland, impatient with schools and bureaucracy, decided to assist them in the project of inclusive schooling. They organised a process of professional development for the teachers of their children which was based upon a dialogical encounter between parents, teachers and administrators.

The overwhelming question emerged from the notion that they were interested in making schools better for all children. Simply put, schools are not so wonderful for the 'normal' kids either. Are we talking about functionalist revisions, or are we grappling with the development of theories of social transformation? Given the evidence that many benefit from the present oppression of disabled children by school education, the task shifts from the theatre of detentes managed through policy accommodations. Integration may in fact be far too great a compromise to make.

The promotion of legitimate alternative identities is more than 'reasonable accommodation'. If we have learned anything from the struggles of women educators it is the necessity of new theories generated through new languages and new social relations established by and not on behalf of oppressed people.

If an agenda for change is to be set, it ought to, as its essential task, enlist schools and their communities in a more careful consideration of disablement. Challenging the conventional special educational wisdom of categorical educational delivery is urgently required. Alternative perspectives should be sought and put by a new group of experts; the disabled, their carers and their advocates. There remains in schools a deep texture of ignorance and mythology about disability which can only be dispelled through such dialogue. Social theories of disability (Swain, Finkelstein, French & Oliver 1993) will provide leadership in the reconstruction of schools committed to inclusion and dissatisfied with tokenistic integration.

To be sure contest and struggle will accompany this enterprise. Resistance from those who preside over the special education industry and integration management is predictable. Parents fearful of threats to the security of their children will also feel considerable discomfiture. The importance of establishing 'inclusion networks' to support parents, students and sympathetic teachers is a tactical requirement (Uditsky 1993).

The status of disability studies in the academies of higher education and teacher training needs to be promoted and brought into the centre of theory debates to inform those who will work in schools in the future (Ainscow 1993). Currently the Australian approach is to give all undergraduate education students core units in special education in order to instruct them in integration. Major research grants in inclusive education continue to be awarded to the traditional special educational research centres which continue to draw their breath from the medical model of disability while exhaling a language of inclusion. This represents the irreconcilability of two discourses and perpetuates the absence of knowledge about disablement in and by schools.

Recruitment in the education departments ought to adhere to equity strategies with respect to the enlistment of disabled educators and researchers in key positions of policy development across the various sites of educational policy making. Aboriginal Australians are appointed to preside over the development of Koori education for all students; multi-cultural education programmes are developed and delivered by people from non-English speaking backgrounds; women lead the reconstruction of schooling to improve the educational outcomes for girls, after first articulating feminist responses to patriarchy. For women's education, policy making was embedded in a theory of education consistent with feminist discourses. We await the reconstruction of schooling according to a disability rights discourse.

References

Abberley, P. (1987) 'The concept of oppression and the development of a social theory of disability', *Disability, Handicap & Society*, 2, 1, pp. 5–19.

Ainscow, M. (1993) 'Teacher education as a strategy for developing inclusive schools' in Slee, R. (ed.) *Is There A Desk With My Name On It? The Politics of Integration*. London: Falmer Press.

American Psychiatric Association (1987) *Diagnostic and Statistical Manual of Mental Disorders*, 3rd Edition. Washington D.C.: APA.

Ball, S. J. (1987) *The Micro-politics of the School*, London, Methuen.

Ball, S. J. (1988) 'Comprehensive schooling, effectiveness and control: an analysis of educational discourses' in Slee, R. (ed.) *Discipline and Schools: A Curriculum Perspective*. Melbourne: Macmillan.

Ball, S. J. (1990a) *Politics and Policy Making in Education: Explorations in Policy Sociology*. London: Routledge.

Ball, S. J. (ed.) (1990b) *Foucault and Education: Discipline and Knowledge*. London: Routledge.

Barkley, R. A. (1990) *Attention Deficit Hyperactivity Disorder: A Handbook for Diagnosis and Treatment*. New York: Guildford Press.

Barnes, C. (1992) 'Qualitative research: valuable or irrelevant?' *Disability, Handicap & Society*, 7, 2, pp. 115–24.

Barton, L. (1987) *The Politics of Special Educational Needs*. Lewes: The Falmer Press.

Barton, L. (1994) 'Disability, difference and the politics of definition' Inaugural Professorial Address to the University of Sheffield, *Australian Disability Review*, September Issue 3.

Bash, L. and Coulby, D. (1989) *The Education Reform Act: Competition and Control*. London: Cassell Educational.

Becker, H. (1963) *The Outsiders*. New York: The Free Press.

Bowe, R. and Ball, S. J. with Gold, A. (1992) *Reforming Education and Changing Schools: Case Studies in Policy Sociology*. London: Routledge.

Bowley, B. A. and Walter, E. (1992) 'Attention deficit disorders and the role of the elementary school counsellor' *Elementary School Guidance and Counselling*, Vol. 27, pp. 39–46.

Branson, J. and Miller, D. (1989) 'Beyond integration policy – the deconstruction of disability' in L. Barton (ed.) *Integration: Myth or Reality*. Lewes: The Falmer Press.

Canter, L. and Canter, M. (1976) *Assertive Discipline: A Take Charge Approach For Today's Educator*. Seals, California: Canter and Associates.

Cohen, S. (1985) *Visions of Social Control*. Cambridge: Polity Press.

Corbett, J. (1994) 'A proud label: exploring the relationship between disability politics and gay pride' *Disability & Society*, 9, 3, pp. 343–57.

de Swann, A. (1990) *The Management of Normality: Critical Essays in Health and Welfare*. London: Routledge.

Edwards, A. (1988) *Regulation and Repression*. Sydney: Allen and Unwin.

Epstein, M. A., Shaywitz, S. E., Shaywitz, B. A. and Woolston, J. L. (1991) 'The boundaries of attention deficit disorder' *Journal of Learning Disabilities, 24*, pp. 78–86.

Finkelstein, V. (1980) *Attitudes and Disabled People: Issues for Discussion*. New York: World Rehabilitation Fund.

Foucault, M. (1979) *Discipline and Punish: The Birth of the Prison*. Harmondsworth: Penguin Books.

Freeland, J. (1992) 'Education and training for the school to work transition', in T. Seddon and C. Deer (eds) *A Curriculum for the Senior Secondary Years*. Hawthorn: Australian Council for Educational Research [ACER].

Fulcher, G. (1987) 'Bureaucracy takes round seven: round eight to commonsense?' *The Age*, Melbourne, April 14.

Fulcher, G. (1989) *Disabling Policies? A comparative approach to education policy and disability*. Lewes: The Falmer Press.

Furlong, V. J. (1985) *The Deviant Pupil*. Milton Keynes: The Open University Press.

Furlong, V. J. (1992) 'Disaffected pupils: reconstructing the sociological perspective' *British Journal of Sociology of Education, 12*, 3, pp. 293–307.

Giroux, H. A. (1992) *Border Crossings*. New York: Routledge.

Glasser, W. (1965) *Reality Therapy*. New York: Harper and Row.

Glasser, W. (1986) *Control Theory In The Classroom*. New York: Harper and Row.

Gordon, T. (1974) *Teacher Effectiveness Training*. New York: Peter H. Wyden.

Govoni, L. E. and Hayes, J. E. (1988) *Drugs and Nursing Implications*. Englewood Cliffs: Prentice-Hall.

Habermas, J. (1976) *Legitimation Crisis*. London: Heinemann.

Hastings, E. (1993) 'Interviewed by Roger Slee' *Australian Disability Review, 1*, pp. 4–13.

Marginson, S. (1993) *Education and Public Policy in Australia*. Cambridge: Cambridge University Press.

Meadmore, D. (1993) 'Divide and rule: a study of two dividing practices in Queensland schools' in R. Slee (ed.) *Is There A Desk With My Name On It? The Politics of Integration*. London: The Falmer Press.

Morris, J. (1992) 'Personal and political: a feminist perspective on researching physical disability' *Disability, Handicap & Society, 7*, 2, pp. 157–66.

Muetzelfeldt, M. and Bates, R. (1992) 'Conflict, contradiction and crisis', in Muetzelfeldt, M. (ed.) *Society, State and Politics in Australia*. Leichhardt: Pluto Press.

Offe, C. (1984) *Contradictions of the Welfare State*. London: Hutchinson.

Oliver, M. (1989) 'Disability and dependency: a creation of industrial societies', in L. Barton (ed.) *Disability and Dependency*. Lewes: The Falmer Press.

Oliver, M. (1990) *The Politics of Disablement*. Basingstoke: Macmillan.

Oliver, M. (1992) 'Changing the social relations of research production?' *Disability, Handicap & Society, 7*, 2, pp. 101–14.

Petersen, A. R. (1994) *In A Critical Condition: Health and Power Relations in Australia.* Sydney: Allen & Unwin.

Polk, K. (1988) 'Education, youth unemployment and student resistance', in R. Slee (ed.) *Discipline and Schools: A Curriculum Perspective.* Melbourne: Macmillan.

Polk, K. and Tait, D. (1990) 'Changing youth labour markets and youth lifestyles' *Youth Studies, 9*, 1, pp. 17–23.

Power, S. (1992) 'Researching the impact of education policy: difficulties and discontinuities' *Journal of Education Policy*, Vol. 7, No. 5, pp. 493–500.

Ramsay, E. (1993) 'Linguistic omissions marginalising women managers', in D. Baker and M. Fogarty (eds) *A Gendered Culture: Educational Management in the Nineties.* Melbourne: Victoria University of Technology.

Rawls, J. (1972) *A Theory of Justice.* Oxford: Oxford University Press.

Rice, M. (1993) 'Integration: another form of specialism', in R. Slee (ed.) *Is There A Desk With My Name On It? The Politics of Integration.* London: The Falmer Press.

Rogers, W. (1989) *Decisive Discipline: Every Move You Make, Every Step You Take* (Video and Workbook Learning Kit). Geelong: Institute of Educational Administration.

Rose, N. (1989) *Governing the Soul: The Shaping of the Private Self.* London: Routledge.

Serfontein, G. (1990) *The Hidden Handicap.* Sydney: Simon & Schuster Australia.

Slee, R. (1993) 'The politics of integration – new sites for old practices?' *Disability, Handicap & Society, 8*, 4, pp. 351–60.

Slee, R. (1995) *Changing Theories and Practices of School Discipline.* London: The Falmer Press.

Smith, D. E. (1988) *The Everyday World as Problematic: a feminist sociology.* Boston: Northeastern University Press.

Swain, J., Finkelstein, V., French, S. and Oliver, M. (1993) (eds) *Disabling Barriers – Enabling Environments.* London: Sage Publications.

Tomlinson, S. (1982) *A Sociology of Special Education.* London: Routledge & Kegan Paul.

Tomlinson, S. (1993) 'Conflicts and dilemmas for professionals in special education' in *Social Justice, Equity and Dilemmas of Disability in Education*, Conference Proceedings – International Working Conference, 1992, Brisbane.

Troyna, B. (1994) 'Blind faith? "empowerment" and educational research', paper presented to the *International Sociology of Education Conference*, Sheffield University.

Troyna, B. (1994) 'Critical social research and education policy', *British Journal of Educational Studies, XXXXII*, 1, pp. 70–84.

Tucker, B. P. (1994) 'Overview of the Disability Discrimination Act [Australia] and comparison with the Americans with Disabilities Act [United States]' *Australian Disability Review*, September, Issue 3.

Uditsky, B. (1993) 'From integration to inclusion: the Canadian experience' in Slee, R. (ed.) *Is There A Desk With My Name On It? The Politics of Integration*. London: The Falmer Press.

Walsh, B. (1993) 'How disabling any handicap is depends on the attitudes and actions of others: a student's perspective', in Slee, R. (ed.) *Is There A Desk With My Name On It? The Politics of Integration*. London: The Falmer Press.

Weiner, G. (1993) 'Feminisms and education in the United Kingdom', seminar presentation to Center for Policy and Leadership Studies, Queensland University of Technology, Kelvin Grove.

White, R. (1990) *No Space Of Their Own: Young People and Social Control in Australia*. Melbourne: Cambridge University Press.

CHAPTER 7

Reflecting on researching disability and higher education

ALAN HURST

This paper attempts to explore some issues associated with undertaking research about how disabled people are involved in higher education in Britain. I see this as an important but neglected social setting in which disabled people continue to encounter oppression. As a sociologist I see it being especially valuable for carrying out the sociological task identified by Len Barton, where it is possible 'to make the connections between structural conditions and the lived reality of people . . .' (Barton 1995; 1).

The paper will consider how much the research can both draw upon existing social theories of disability and contribute to their further development. It begins with a brief personal statement in which I identify the situation I find myself in and the kinds of questions I am facing. This is followed by an outline of current policy and provision for disabled people in higher education. Having laid these foundations it becomes possible to indicate some problems facing those pursuing research and also how policies and practices at institutional and national levels might be linked to theories. The paper ends with sóme thoughts about future action.

A personal history

I feel it is necessary to include some details of my personal history and contemporary situation since I share the feelings about my research interests and involvements identified by Barton:

What right have I to undertake this work?
What responsibilities arise from the privileges I have as a result of my social position?

I would like to thank Sharon Clancy, Martin Pagel and Judith Russell of the Sheffield Hallam University HEFC(E) Project for the inspiration behind these personal reflections.

How can I use my knowledge and skills to challenge the forms of oppression disabled people experience and thereby help to empower them?
Does my writing and speaking reproduce a system of domination or challenge that system?
Have I shown respect to the disabled people I have worked with?

(Barton 1994:10)

Unlike some of the contributors to this book I do not have a disability. I have a sight defect and have worn spectacles to correct this since I was three years old. I know too that with age the defect is becoming more serious. Also I take regular and frequent medication to control attacks of migraine. Although I was subjected to taunting as a child ('specky four-eyes' etc.) and although I am made aware that some people feel that migraine can be equated to having a severe headache I cannot claim to have experienced the hostility, prejudice and oppression felt by others.

In my professional life, having obtained a first degree in history and sociology, I spent some time teaching in mainstream secondary education before becoming involved in higher education. As my experience grew and my responsibilities widened to eventually encompass the role of undergraduate admissions tutor for a combined studies degree programme I became aware of the very small number of applications from people who made it clear that they had disabilities. Later I was able to explore this in more detail (Hurst 1990; Hurst 1993). Meanwhile I had become involved with the actual development of provision for disabled students in my own institution and I had become a member of the National Bureau for Handicapped Students. This organisation had emerged as a result of a meeting of educationists, other professionals and some students in November 1974. The initiative for this meeting originated in a conference held the previous year in which it was suggested that many suitably qualified young people could not take advantages of opportunities offered by higher education since the facilities and support services they needed were not available. Since those early days the organisation has grown although its basic aim to develop opportunities in post-compulsory education for all students irrespective of impairment or learning difficulty remains the same. In 1988 the charity changed its name to Skill: National Bureau for Students with Disabilities to reflect changes in attitude and language. As time has passed I have continued my work with disabled students in my own institution and have taken on responsibilities within Skill. At the time of writing I convene its national Higher Education Working Party and act as the organisation's Senior Vice-Chair. This means that I have a significant responsibility within a national charity alongside those associated with my roles at my university. I am also a member of the group set up by the Higher Education Funding Council (England) following its creation by the Further and Higher Education Act 1992 and complying with the guidance from the Secretary of State that the situation of disabled students should be the focus of some attention. (Further details about this group are given later.) Within the group it is intended that I offer informed advice concerning policies and provision relating to disabled students in higher education. My membership of this group presents the chance to influence policy at national level.

This brief resumé of my own circumstances helps explain some of the questions and dilemmas I face both as a sociologist interested in researching this sector of educational provision and as an individual keen to ensure that disabled people have the same opportunities and rights as everyone else.

Returning to those questions posed by Len Barton and responding to them, I want to point out that:

(a) as a non-disabled person I have grown increasingly aware of the issues surrounding my 'right' to undertake the work I do;

(b) as a senior member of a national charity and of a potentially influential national policy-oriented group I experience dilemmas about my responsibilities;

(c) again following from the above I am concerned that what I do leads to the ending of oppression and the growth of empowerment within both higher education and society;

(d) my roles have involved me in taking up more opportunities to speak in public and to write about disability issues in higher education; in doing so I hope that I avoid reproducing the status quo;

(e) I am anxious that my work with disabled students and disabled colleagues is conducted in ways which they feel are appropriate and acceptable.

Having made my own position clearer I must now give an outline of the national educational context of my work.

Higher education and disabled people

Sociological research on learners with disabilities and learning difficulties has neglected the higher education sector. It could be argued also that the issues raised in higher education are ignored in the comments of colleagues. Thus Slee, having urged caution in talking in general terms about the experience of disability, continues to discuss issues of inclusion in 'education' when his concern appears to be with compulsory schooling only (Slee 1995). In fact, in relation to debates about inclusive education, the situation in higher education in Britain is that the basic notion of segregation and discrete provision is absent. Instead the 'inclusion' debate relates more to physical difficulties posed by the environment, technical difficulties relating to accessing the curriculum, and extra-curricular difficulties about living accommodation and social life.

Compared to some countries, most obviously the USA, little is known about disabled people in higher education in the UK. It should be noted that I have chosen to use the word 'people' here since I want to draw attention to the fact that my concern is not only with disabled students but also with disabled staff. This neglect can be identified in two respects: research and policy.

In terms of research in Britain, until recently there was little information available about disabled people in higher education and what there is almost entirely concerned with students. Arguably the most significant quantitative investigation was that sponsored by the National Innovations Centre and published in 1974 (NIC 1974). Questionnaires were sent to 150 institutions but only 53 responded. Perhaps the low rate of return is indicative of the lack of concern felt at that time. However, based on responses from 242 individuals, the findings are reported under ten headings: student profile (age, sex, schooling, disability), entry to higher education, academic life, books and libraries, examinations, getting about, accommodation, health and welfare, social life, and jobs. In all sections the information is presented in tabular form with linking analysis and commentary. Another survey with a similar statistically oriented approach was published in 1987 although this was concerned only with public sector provision (i.e. the polytechnics) and did not examine universities. What was missing from studies like these was an indication of the lived experiences of the disabled students. This is what I tried to incorporate into my own work with some small groups of students with impaired mobility (Hurst 1993). I tried also to set the students' experiences within the context of both institutional and national policies. However, the investigation was inadequate on several counts. It looked only at the circumstances impinging upon students with one kind of impairment and it looked mainly at the process of admission. Whether blind students or deaf students share similar experiences or what the total experience of undergraduate life is was not explored. To some extent the investigation was also overtaken by important national policy developments relating to funding.

As with other sectors of the education service higher education has undergone considerable changes since the coming to power of the series of Conservative administrations. The nature of the changes has been summarised recently: 'At the same time higher education is changing: from provider to market . . . different learners . . . expansion . . . different learning . . . flexibility . . . partnership . . .'

(NIACE 1994:1)

Within these changes the situation of disabled students has been given some consideration. From the perspective of the individual student the financial position has improved since 1990. In that year the government introduced a system of top-up loans for students. As a result of pressure from many quarters concerned that the system might cause additional financial hardship for disabled students, the government modified the existing disabled students awards. (For details on how the pressures were applied see Hurst 1993.) Disabled students who qualify for a maintenance award from their local education authorities can apply for three additional allowances to cover the costs incurred as a direct result of the disability, the costs of any special equipment, and the costs of non-medical personal help with study. The amount of money available each year has been increased in line with the rate of inflation. Without doubt the additional allowances have been valuable. However, there are problems which remain to be addressed – for example, the exclusion of part-time students and the varying procedures adopted by different local education authorities (see Patton 1990).

Whilst many students have benefited, the problems faced by the institutions themselves were not addressed. In fact much of the literature published at the turn of the decade which concerned widening access and improving the participation rates of certain disadvantaged groups ignored disabled people (Hurst 1992). Although some universities, polytechnics and colleges were developing policies and provision, the majority were doing nothing. If challenged about this the most frequent responses cited costs to explain their lack of action. Certainly there was no incentive to spend money on adapting facilities or employing appropriate staff since the institutions were not given additional allowances for this work. Perhaps, too, the activities of the small minority which were making progress acted as a disincentive since it appeared things were being done already by others. The major change came following the Further and Higher Education Act 1992 which introduced a unified system of control and finance for the entire sector. Again further pressure was put on government and in his guidance to the newly created national funding councils the Secretary of State for Education insisted that they gave particular attention to meeting the needs of disabled people.

The response of the English Funding Council was to establish an Advisory Group on Widening Participation. From the first meeting it was clear that there was a concern to support developments for disabled students. It announced that for the academic year 1993–4 £3m was being set aside as a Special

Initiative. Institutions were invited to bid for finance to support their own projects, funding being allocated by the Advisory Group according to criteria published in the circular encouraging bids. Over 100 applications were made and had all been supported the total cost would have been £8.2m. The Advisory Group tried to adjudicate in terms of projects which built upon existing good practice and experience and which could act as exemplars for the sector. The money was not intended to support projects which were based on very limited experience. It was also made clear that the funds were to act as a pump-priming strategy and that the institutions should consider how the projects could be embedded into their working practices. In total, 38 projects were supported covering policies and provision for working with students with a range of disabilities. The Initiative is being evaluated and an interim report about the first year has already been published (HEFCE 1995). Even before the end of the first year the Funding Council announced that it had allocated a second tranche of £3m for 1994–5 and this time 49 projects have been supported. (At this point it should be noted that the Funding Councils for Scotland and for Wales have taken action to encourage the development of policies and provision but their strategies have been different from what has happened in England.)

It is against this background that the rest of this paper is set. However, I must reiterate that I would like to include disabled staff as well as students in the discussion and analysis. It should be evident already that the former are very much an 'invisible' group in any work that has been undertaken so far. I think that there might be several very important reasons for this. Many academic staff working in post-compulsory education are qualified teachers, some of whom have had experience working in schools. In order to obtain a place on an initial teacher-training course applicants have to be deemed to be medically fit. This is where the difficulties arise. Some people with disabilities have had medical examinations after which the doctor has indicated that they are 'fit' to teach; others have been defined as 'unfit' on the grounds of their disability. This is a major cause for concern and an area of negative discrimination which the Royal Association for Disability and Rehabilitation is pursuing (RADAR 1993). In particular attempts are being made to change the intrusive and offensive questionnaire which disabled applicants have to complete. Because of these barriers there might be fewer disabled qualified teaching staff in higher education – hence their 'invisibility'.

A second contributory cause relates to qualifications. In order to teach in higher education tutors are usually expected to be well qualified and to have themselves been students in higher education. Higher education is important in giving people the qualifications and credentials necessary for future employment. Abberley has drawn attention to the denial of employment opportunities for disabled people (Abberley 1995). Whilst this might be a reflection of prejudice, it might also be linked to the denial of opportunities to disabled people to obtain the necessary qualifications. As I have suggested already if disabled people are an under-represented group in the student population in higher education, this might be replicated within both the general labour market and also amongst the academic employees of universities.

There are no figures available about the number of disabled teachers working in higher education, nor are there any for disabled employees in general in our universities. Universities may hold attitudes similar to those found most commonly amongst employers. In early 1995 the government introduced a parliamentary bill to end discrimination against disabled people. The accompanying White Paper states that higher education in England is to be the subject of a review, although the implication is that it will be considered from the perspective of students rather than employees (HMSO 1995).

Perhaps a more constructive solution for both potential staff and students is to introduce a more active process of disability awareness raising in the institutions. However, in doing so, there are several important questions to be addressed. Firstly, there are questions about who should be involved both as recipients and as deliverers. There are arguments suggesting that everybody in an institution, from the most senior to the most junior and irrespective of their work responsibilities, should participate in awareness-raising programmes. To some extent the difficulty with this is the scale of the enterprise. Also, those who have attempted this comment consistently that those who appear to be in greatest need are the ones who seldom attend. A compromise approach involves the targeting of particular groups – for example, the course team responsible for a subject where disabled students have enrolled or those working in a disabled students' hall of residence. In considering who should organise disability awareness-raising programmes, those who have introduced programmes into their own institutions have demonstrated a strong commitment to employing groups and organisations of disabled people. A point to consider here is the extent to which those delivering the sessions have both the experience and the training for the task.

A second set of questions relates to the timing of disability awareness raising. One strategy is to provide it prior to the first contact with a disabled person, whilst another is to postpone it until later so that those about to have their awareness raised are already facing up to some important issues. Each has its strengths and weaknesses but there is one aspect on which there is total agreement – awareness raising means much more than organising single events. It has to be a continuous activity with a clearly defined programme. One way in which this might be accomplished is to ensure that it has a place in the induction of all those new to the institution. Staff development/personnel sections might take on the responsibility for employees whilst student unions ought to play a major part in raising the awareness of their members. Also in addition to the formal approach, there are many other opportunities to draw attention to disability issues, for example staff and student research projects, and attention at course validation and review events.

A third series of questions deals with the content and methods of disability awareness-raising programmes. There is an increasing amount of commercially produced material available, although this might benefit from altering and amending to suit the particular context of the institution. In the past, there has been an approach based on simulation exercises, but this has been the subject of some debate (see French 1992). What also merits attention is the issue of whether what is being provided is about 'educating' participants or whether it constitutes 'training'.

Researching disability in higher education: some issues

In view of my previous comment I hope that it is understandable that I will direct my comments towards undertaking research involving disabled students. I must begin by trying to define 'disabled' student and giving some indication of who might be involved.

At the outset it needs to be made clear that there are no figures available giving precise statistical information about the number of disabled students involved in higher education. This situation is about to change since the recently created Higher Education Statistics Agency (HESA) will be collecting information about disability as part of its regular practices. In the absence of such information deriving from the institutions and published centrally it is possible to obtain some overall picture based on the information given to the organisations responsible for coordinating the majority of applications for places in higher education institutions at the point of application. (Prior to the unifying of the higher education system following the Further and Higher Education Act 1992 there were two organisations involved: the Universities Central Council on Admissions and the Polytechnics Central Admissions System; since 1992 the procedures have been taken over by a single body, the Universities and Colleges Admissions Service.) Prior to 1992 individual applicants were asked to indicate if they had a disability by simply ticking a box. They were not required to give additional information. (See Cooper (1990) for an analysis based on subject choices and acceptance rates.) The system posed a dilemma for many since they felt that by indicating their disability their application would be rejected. Following pressure from Skill and other organisations, the system was changed so that the standard UCAS application form now asks all applicants to complete a particular section of the form in which a range of disabilities can be indicated. The accompanying guidance notes stress that providing such information is intended to help institutions make appropriate provision in advance of entry to the course. On the basis of responses to the categories of disability it is possible now to gain a clearer picture of the number of disabled applicants and their disabilities. (Note that the focus is on applications rather than on actual entry to higher education.) The categories provide an 'official' definition of disability within the context of higher education. They cover the following: specific learning difficulty (e.g. dyslexia), partial sight and blindness, partial hearing and deafness, mobility difficulties and wheelchair users, students needing personal assistance, mental health difficulties, unseen disabilities, and multiple disabilities.

Of the above the largest number of students claim to have some form of specific learning difficulty, usually dyslexia. Confirmation of dyslexia as a major concern for higher education institutions is provided also by the predominance of project applications submitted to the HEFCE Advisory Group on Widening Participation. Further comment and also information about specific projects is provided in the report on the 1993–4 Special Initiative (HEFCE 1995). The considerable rise in the number of students has presented many problems. After submitting written work which is deemed to be unsatisfactory in some way, some students suspect for the first time that they have dyslexia. In order to have this confirmed officially they must have an assessment by a qualified educational psychologist. This then leads to the question of how the assessment is paid for. If the dyslexia is confirmed students can then apply for the additional financial support available through the Disabled Students Awards (DSA) to pay for the educational psychologist's recommendations and to buy equipment. However, as the possibility of securing more funding, especially for the purchase of personal computers, has become better known and as the nature of a specific learning difficulty can be used to try to mask weaknesses in study skills, it appears that more students are putting themselves forward for assessment. The consequences of this have been to overload the staff working to support disabled students in the institutions and a growing scepticism on the part of local education authority awards officers in the face of the huge increase in applications for the DSA. In addition to these issues of identification and assessment there are matters relating to the academic side of higher education which have to be addressed. For example, some institutions offer additional tutorial support which is not subject specific and is intended to assist students with their learning difficulties. The extent of this support and what it should consist of poses some questions relating to the originality and ownership of written work submitted for formal assessment. Without doubt an important impact of the HEFCE Special Initiatives has been to stimulate debate about specific learning difficulties.

Having tried to identify those who might be regarded as disabled students I can address a number of other issues. Many of these stem from the view that any research must allow the subjects to speak for themselves. In my experience of working with disabled students this has not been an easy task. Firstly, many disabled students see being a student as being the more significant experience. This is akin to the issues highlighted by Barton when noting the situation of disabled women and black disabled people. To paraphrase his comment, disabled students mediate their experiences within the context of being a university student and 'these compound the oppressions involved' (Barton 1995:7). Thus for many disabled students their major concerns are with more general issues affecting all students – the cost of living, meeting work deadlines, having a good social life. For most full-time undergraduates being a student is a fleeting, transient experience; in the first year they undergo a process of resocialisation, in the second year they enjoy their new life, and in the third and final years they focus on exams, graduation and getting a job. Perhaps the negative perceptions of students in general also 'rub off' on disabled students. Consequently, many disabled students whose views and experiences could contribute significantly to an investigation prefer not to become involved. They wish to play down their disabilities. Putting this differently and indicating a related issue they can perhaps be regarded as 'students with disabilities' rather than 'disabled students'. It is interesting that this is a point I commented upon in the introduction to my own investigation (Hurst 1993) and which has been raised again more recently in connection with developing policy in Australia (National Board of Education, Employment and Training 1994). A final point to note is that within the group of disabled students there are important differences. Thus deaf students sometimes wish to develop a community of their own based on their own culture and language (see the comments below concerning the Sheffield Hallam University project). This is quite different from the approach of other groups seeking a closer involvement and inclusion in student life. As stated earlier the largest group of students in higher education consists of those with specific learning difficulties rather than those with what might be more commonly regarded as disabilities. The point I am making here is that any research should try to identify both the concerns relevant to all disabled students and those specific to a particular group.

Having overcome some of the difficulties of involving disabled students in research the next stage is to consider methods. My own preference is for qualitative approaches and so this prompts questions about data collection using interviews, observations and documentary sources. I have said already that I do not have a disability and so in any interviews with disabled students I cannot claim to be what Goffman termed one of 'the own'. This could create barriers and difficulties. In terms of reporting any findings I am aware too of the need to let the students speak for themselves (Booth, Chapter 12 of this volume). My own preference would be to try to incorporate into my work the three postulates identified by Alfred Schutz. Schutz was used by David Hargreaves in his investigation of deviant behaviour in schools (Hargreaves 1975). In outlining his approach Hargreaves comments:

There are two basic problems for the social scientist: the discovery of the first order constructs of the members that are relevant to the scientific problem, and the translation of these into second order constructs that comprise the scientific theory. In relation to the second Schutz (1953) offers three postulates which specify the requirements that must be fulfilled by scientific concepts.

(Hargreaves 1975:27–30)

The first postulate, the postulate of logical consistency, is concerned with logic and the ways in which the basis of knowledge used by the investigator differs from the basis of knowledge of his subjects. In short it is the difference between scientific knowledge and common-sense knowledge. One way in which this can be brought to notice is for the views of the subjects, in this case disabled students, to be reported verbatim alongside any analysis and discussion arising from them. In reality this might not be feasible when a researcher has accumulated transcripts of many interviews. The second postulate, the postulate of subjective interpretation, emphasises the importance of the researcher giving recognition to perspectives of the individual when discussing social actions. It is the meaning of the situation for the subject which is important, not that of the researcher. The third postulate, the postulate of adequacy, is about the extent to which the researcher's analysis and interpretation of actions is understood by and accords with the views of those being researched. Pursuing this would mean that, prior to reporting, those involved as the subjects of the investigation should be allowed to comment on what is being proposed. Thus, the disabled students would need to confirm or amend my proposed version of the situation. Again, this might be impractical for many reasons, not least of which might be time.

At this point we are starting to encompass a discussion of the relationship of methodology to theory. As has been noted elsewhere, research about disability has been notable for its atheoretical approach, although Shakespeare has noted the development of social theories of disability since 1980 (Shakespeare 1994). This lack of articulation with theory is evident in research on disability and higher education. Certainly there is an absence in such research which treats seriously the perspectives of disabled students. Perhaps this results from a lack of readily available, easy-to-use theories on the one hand or, on the other hand, an inability to employ C. Wright Mills's 'sociological imagination'. However there are indications that some progress is being made. What is also notable is the linking of theory to practice.

Linking theory, policy and practice: a case study

Mention has been made already of the projects funded by the HEFCE Special Initiative. One of the 38 successful bids in 1993–4 came from Sheffield Hallam University, the intention being to undertake a systematic audit of what the University had available to support disabled students and how the development of a new framework could enhance provision. The project encouraged the close involvement of disabled people, mainly students but also a small group of disabled staff. It was built upon a two key principles. Firstly, it made a clear statement about the social model of disability and the social oppression resulting from this. Whilst many other projects and many other institutions subscribe to and uphold this view, the project team at Sheffield Hallam gave it great emphasis. Secondly, the project team was keen to recognise disability culture. Within this the importance of the experience of disability, self definition, self determination, and self advocacy were acknowledged. On this foundation the team tried to develop a system rooted in a social theory of disability. The team took as its starting point the principles of independent living identified by disabled people and applied them to the context of higher education. The definition of 'independence' is concerned with the extent to which disabled people/students are in control of their own lives and are able to organise them in the ways that they want. Also important is the idea of 'choice' – being able to decide for themselves. Again many universities recognise this although often this is more implicit than explicit.

The first of the seven principles is about information and access to it. Thus, for blind students, materials should be available in a format which they desire. For some this will mean in braille; for others pre-recorded cassettes are the preferred medium. For students with other kinds of visual impairment, providing materials in large print is necessary. Access to information is also a matter which concerns deaf students. For example, information should be made available through the use of British Sign Language. No matter what the nature of the disability, the concern here is with the total 'information environment'. It is very easy to assume that what is at stake is access to the formal curriculum. However, what disabled students have the right to is information about the total student experience and in the format that they want. Thus, at the initial stage of admissions, an institution's prospectus should be produced in different formats. If a university produces a video to attract students the commentary should reassure blind viewers that they are not missing important information transmitted in the pictures. Equally the video should have either subtitles or a signed commentary on a part of the picture. Once on course, not only is there 'academic' information, there is also the plethora of news about events and happenings in the social life of the university. How will blind students find out about the visit of a leading politician if this is advertised on flyers placed on tables in the bar? How will deaf students know that the time of the event has had to be changed at the last minute if the information is conveyed only by the public address in the student union building? These are not major problems. They do not involve expensive technology. They can be eliminated if the community is made aware of the rights of disabled students and takes steps to ensure that these are not denied. This point links closely with the issues of awareness raising discussed earlier.

The second principle relates to peer support. The experiences of other disabled students can be of considerable benefit if they can be shared with others. At this point I must refer to something mentioned earlier – some (many?) disabled students do not wish to be identified with their disability and so choose not to become involved in ensuring that their university does not deny them their rights. The Sheffield Hallam project made great efforts to gain the involvement of disabled students. In particular an introductory programme was devised to try to encourage participation from disabled students as soon as they joined the University. Following this, the project team has published a short report offering the views of those who took part (Sheffield Hallam University 1994). One intention is that the early involvement will lead to more participation in the existing Disabled Students Forum. An interesting aspect of this – and one which again relates back to a comment made earlier – is that deaf students have formed their own 'splinter group'. A danger with developments such as this is the divisiveness of the experience.

The third principle of independent living concerns housing. As with almost all other universities, there is a shortage of accessible and affordable accommodation. Many universities have developed adapted living accommodation, especially in their halls of residence. However, the costs of living there are expensive and some students cannot afford the rents. For some students this may be the only possibility and yet by choice they would like to live with friends in flats, or rented houses. An alternative might be to attend a university near to home and so continue to live with parents, but this might deny the opportunity to leave home which many people welcome. The Sheffield Hallam team recognise the right to live where the individual chooses. To this end they suggest that universities could try to become more influential in their approaches to local authorities and to housing associations to ensure that a range of suitable accommodation is available in the local area.

Moving to the fourth principle, technical aids, the Sheffield Hallam team affirm the right of disabled students to equipment which they need. At this point it is possible to draw attention again to the additional financial allowances introduced in 1990 and to the shortcomings of the system. Some students do not qualify for this support either because they are part-time or because the application of the means test on their parents' income has debarred them. Secondly, for some students, the money available is insufficient. For example, if a deaf student employs a communicator in her/his classes, the cost per hour is approximately £15. Assuming the communicator works for ten hours each week this student faces a bill of £150 per week or £1500 per term. The non-medical personal assistance allowance is currently £4750 and so over the period of an academic year a deaf student might use almost the entire allowance on this support alone. Some universities do offer access to equipment in different ways. For example, some have bursaries which allow students to purchase necessary items whilst others have a stock of items which they lend to students for the duration of their course. One important point noted by the Sheffield Hallam team is the availability of independent, informed advice about equipment appropriate to an individual's needs. Whilst recognising this, in terms of the earlier definition of 'independence', a disabled student is free to ignore any advice. Buying specific items might not be compulsory although, for example, if IT equipment has been chosen because of its compatibility with a university's system, ignoring advice could create difficulties. However, the key to equipment is its function in supporting a disabled student to achieve maximum independence.

In addition to equipment some disabled students need personal assistants. Trying to meet the needs of disabled students has involved many different universities in a variety of schemes. Some choose to use Community Service Volunteers whilst others have appointed their own staff specifically for this work. For the Sheffield Hallam team the only solution in accordance with the principles of independent living is one where the disabled student has direct control over those who are providing the assistance. The personal assistants become the employees of the individual and are there to do those things for which there is no other means available.

The sixth principle is about the environment. In order to achieve independence, disabled students have the right to access all facilities. In many universities this is possible since a gradual programme of conversions and adaptations have met the needs of disabled people. However, there are many problems. Thus, whilst access to buildings is possible, it is not always via the most direct, most convenient or most generally used routes. Also, in higher education, geography and architecture present other barriers. Many buildings occupied by the older universities have listed status and so any plans to improve access are met with considerable caution. The newer universities were often campus based rather than city-centre sites and thus the layout of the campus is significant. The former polytechnics are often based on several sites and this also creates difficulties.

The final principle of independent living used by the Sheffield Hallam Project team concerns transport. They note that disabled people have a right to accessible, affordable public transport. This becomes significant when considering both inter-site travel within institutions and travelling to the nearby town when based at a campus university. There is considerable evidence about the lack of access to public transport in this country. In 1993 London Transport made great publicity out of the fact that they had 'opened' the Underground system to more disabled people and especially to wheelchair users. In truth, of the 270 stations only about 40 are totally accessible and of these very few are in central London. On the main railway system British Rail are moving only slowly to improve access to the network for disabled users. On buses more attention is being given to access for blind and visually impaired passengers although in only a very small number of locations are bus services totally accessible to wheelchair users. (This will change if the proposals in the government's 1995 White Paper become enshrined in law.) In the USA the University of Illinois has gained a reputation for its policies and provision for disabled students. Whilst the importance of civil rights legislation has to be acknowledged it is also the presence of a large number of disabled students in the Champagne-Urbana area that has led to the improvements in the district's transport system. All buses are accessible to wheelchair users and so they can travel where and when they want. In England totally accessible public transport is in its infancy although it is interesting to point out that disabled staff working at Sheffield Hallam University have been involved in the design and development of Sheffield's new rapid transit system.

To me a major value of the approach adopted by the Sheffield Hallam project is that by using the concept of independence it offers the possibility of using a theoretically oriented approach to those investigating issues of disability as they impinge upon participation in higher education. It becomes possible to consider aspects of general policy and provision and also specific component parts (e.g. admissions procedures, accommodation policies) using a schema based around a social model of disability. What is equally important is that the framework offered has its origins amongst disabled people themselves.

Some further reflections

The two recent initiatives sponsored by the Higher Education Funding Council (England) and their parallels in Scotland (see SHEFC 1994) and Wales have done much to project disability on to institutional agendas. It will be interesting to see the extent to which the momentum brought about by the Funding Councils continues and especially so after 1995 when the second special initiative ends. What is not clear at this early stage is whether the projects have actually increased the number of disabled students in higher education or whether they have acted to improve the quality of the experience for the existing group of students. In future, statistics collected by the Higher Education Statistics Agency will address the former whilst the latter ought to be a major concern for the various quality assurance and quality monitoring bodies created alongside the Funding Councils.

No matter what the outcome, the issue of finance will remain. Currently there appears to be a number of strategies directed towards ensuring that institutions do not feel that they are incurring a self-inflicted financial penalty when choosing to spend money on developing policies and provision for disabled students. One approach is to create an enhanced tariff for students with disabilities so that no matter where they go to study they take with them a premium rate of funding. Whilst this has the appeal of not impinging upon student choice, there appear to be no guarantees that the funds will be used to the benefit of the disabled student. At its extreme an unscrupulous institution could set out deliberately to recruit disabled students only for the additional funds they might bring with them. One of the Special Initiative projects funded in 1994–5 is actually investigating tariff-based funding of disabled students.

A second strategy is that currently operational in Australia. In brief this involves institutions in producing equity plans which indicate ways in which they will improve access and support. Once this has been undertaken the institution is reimbursed for the money it has spent on carrying out the work. A problem with this scheme is that it might involve institutions in heavy expenditure from their own resources prior to obtaining retrospective funding.

A recent policy document from Australia has indicated a strategy for development which would be unacceptable, especially in terms of the earlier discussion of the nature of 'independence'. The 'Guidelines for Disability Services in Higher Education' state:

It would not be possible, physically or financially, for each higher education institution in Australia to provide the whole range of special services and facilities identified as necessary or desirable in this report. Because of this, it is reasonable for institutions to consider a degree of specialisation, so that effort, personnel, equipment and experience may be concentrated to achieve the maximum result. Such specialisation could be coordinated within a locality . . .

(National Board of Employment, Education and Training 1994:x)

This 'centres of excellence' approach is not new. One can see its appeal to a number of constituencies. Accountants might favour it on grounds of cost effectiveness and efficiency, and some disabled students might like it because they know in advance that an institution has had previous experience of working with students with the same disability. What this approach does not do is allow the same opportunities and choices to disabled people as it does to others. For this reason such proposals should be resisted. It is the policy of Skill: National Bureau for Students with Disabilities to resist such proposals and in my current role as Senior Vice-Chair of the organisation it presents no dilemma for me since my personal and professional views and the views of the members of the organisation I represent coincide. However, this does lead into a discussion of another issue relevant to this paper – the role of charities.

Skill is a small national charity. It was established in 1974 and since then where the focus was very much on higher education, it has become involved with all aspects of education and training in the post-compulsory sector. The organisation consists of an elected Governing Council whose members represent different interest groups and which decides the organisation's policies, a small elected Executive Committee which is responsible for ensuring that the Governing Council's decisions are put into practice, and a small complement of full-time paid staff who carry out the policies. There are several aspects of Skill and my roles within it which need further discussion.

To begin with I am aware of the debates and concerns that exist about organisations 'of' and organisations 'for' disabled people. Currently Skill is closer to the latter although a more appropriate description might be that it is an organisation 'of and for' disabled people. In 1995 four of the nine members of the Executive Committee declared a disability. Members of Skill do make considerable efforts to encourage the participation of disabled people, especially students. That it does so with only moderate success is a problem. Some of the difficulties result from the aspects of student life outlined earlier. Other matters can be linked to the cost of attending regular meetings in London and to the difficulties of using public transport. Perhaps, too, whilst the organisation appears to be dominated by non-disabled professionals like me, disabled students are put off closer involvement. I (and many of my colleagues in Skill) recognise this as a major issue.

A second point is related to the above. In Chapter 8 Robert Drake is very critical of charities, especially for their lack of disabled representation, for their narrow focus and for contributing towards the status quo and the perpetuation of a medical model of disability. I would wish to take issue with him in relation to Skill. Already I have acknowledged the level of participation by disabled people (especially students) as an issue. However, in terms of focus, Skill works alongside people with a range of disabilities and learning difficulties and so does not fit the model of charities on which he bases his argument. Skill's major concern is to remove the barriers to participation for all disabled people in post-compulsory education. In making this its aim it is adopting a social model of disability and one which recognises the rights of individuals.

The charity has found itself in some interesting situations. Like all charities it depends for much of its income on donations and grants. Some years ago a short appeal was broadcast on BBC television. At the start of filming script ideas originating with the television producers emphasised the 'triumph over tragedy' angle of the participation of disabled students in post-compulsory education. This led to a series of negotiations about how the film should present images of disabled students. Those people working with Skill demanded that the image should be one of independence. Eventually this approach prevailed, although the media team felt that projecting an image which would please disabled people would not at the same time cause people to want to make donations. I think this example demonstrates that Skill's intention is to change the system rather than the individual.

A third point concerns Skill's potential to influence policy in higher education. In recent times persuasive argument from those associated with Skill has contributed to the changes to the standard application form and to the improved financial position of many disabled students. Following the directive from the Secretary of State for Education and the creation of the HEFCE Advisory Group on Widening Participation Skill was invited to join the group to offer advice and comment about disabled students in higher education. After some discussion it was suggested that I should become the representative on the Advisory Group. This has led me to some critical reflections and to considering my responsibilities. In particular I worry about my role as a potential instigator of change. In the background I am aware of the writings of disabled activists such as Paul Abberley and Mike Oliver who are critical of the structural barriers and who as disabled people themselves experience the oppression that I do not. In order to placate them perhaps my contribution to the workings of the HEFCE Group should be more radical. I should be advocating a new 'higher education'. On the other hand, I am aware of the imperatives of the status quo and that changes can also be brought about by a more gradual approach which might be described as liberal rather than radical. Hence I have welcomed the two Special Initiatives, the additional money they have brought and the additional attention that has been directed towards disability in their wake. The bids from the institutions themselves indicate the inadequacy of £6m. On the other hand, if the projects funded have provided additional opportunities and ensured that there are more disabled students in our universities, an important step forward has been made.

Conclusions

Higher education and disability is an important arena, especially in terms of potential for change. When disabled people enter higher education they are taking up an opportunity to increase their knowledge, to develop their social skills, to obtain good qualifications and to expose themselves to debate and discussion. It is an important experience for empowerment. Upon graduation, hopefully they will enter the world of employment and make a potentially important contribution to the disability movement. This process is more advanced than ever before in the United Kingdom. What would make this more effective and thereby make a stronger contribution to disability rights campaigns would be for disabled students and the small number of disabled staff to work together. An alliance of disabled students and disabled teachers could do much to re-educate us and to raise our awareness. In doing so, in Marx's terms, they would be moving from a 'class in itself' to a 'class for itself' and would be a valuable force in the drive for empowerment not just of themselves but of all disabled people.

References

Abberley, P. (1995) 'Work, utopia and impairment' Chapter 4 of this volume.

Barton, L. (1994) 'Disability, difference and the politics of definition' *Australian Disability Review* 3–94 pp. 8–22.

Barton, L. (1995) 'Sociology and disability: some emerging issues' Chapter 1 of this volume.

Cooper, D. (1990) 'University entrance for students with disabilities' unpublished paper. London: Skill.

Drake, R. (1995) 'The exercise of power in the voluntary sector'. Chapter 8 of this volume.

French, S. (1992) 'Simulation exercises in disability awareness training: a critique' *Disability, Handicap & Society*, Vol. 7, No. 3, pp. 257–66.

Hargreaves, D. *et al.* (1975) *Deviance in Classrooms*. London: Routledge & Kegan Paul.

Higher Education Funding Council for England (HEFCE) (1995) *Access to Higher Education: Students with Special Needs – An HEFCE Report on the 1993–94 Special Initiative to Encourage Widening Participation for Students with Special Needs*. Bristol: HEFCE.

HMSO (1995) *Ending Discrimination Against Disabled People*. London: HMSO.

Hurst, A. (1990) 'Obstacles to overcome: higher education and disabled students' in J. Corbett (ed.) *Uneasy Transitions: Disaffection in Post-Compulsory Education*. Basingstoke: Falmer Press.

Hurst, A. (1992) 'Widening participation in higher education and people with disabilities' *Personnel Review*, Vol. 21, No. 6, pp. 19–36.

Hurst, A. (1993) *Steps Towards Graduation: Access to Higher Education for People with Disabilities*. Aldershot: Avebury.

National Board of Education, Employment and Training (1994) *Guidelines for Disability Services in Higher Education*. Canberra: Australian Government Publishing Services.

National Innovations Centre (NIC) (1974) *Disabled Students in Higher Education*. London: NIC.

National Institute for Adult and Continuing Education (1994) *An Adult Higher Education: A Vision*. Leicester: NIACE.

Patton, B. (1990) 'A survey of the Disabled Students Allowances' *Educare* No. 36 (March 1990 pp. 3–7).

Royal Association for Disability and Rehabilitation (RADAR) (1993) *So You Want to be a Teacher?*. London: RADAR.

Scottish Higher Education Funding Council (SHEFC) (1994) *Access to Success for Students with Disabilities in Higher Education in Scotland.* Edinburgh: SHEFC.

Shakespeare, T. (1994) 'Cultural reproduction of disabled people: dustbins for disavowal' *Disability & Society*, Vol. 9, No. 3, pp. 283–301.

Sheffield Hallam University (1994) *Follow the Yellow Brick Road.* Sheffield: Sheffield Hallam University.

Slee, R. (1995) 'Clauses of conditionality: the "reasonable" accommodation of language' Chapter 6 of this volume.

PART THREE

Disability, Charities, Normalisation and Representation

How disability is defined is of crucial importance. This involves several factors including our past experience of interacting with disabled people, as well as the impact of the images depicted through a range of mass-media outlets.

Many such images are negative, often based on medical assumptions and unexamined views of normality. These contribute to a dependency-creating culture in which professional and official definitions and decisions on behalf of disabled people become part of the accepted ethos.

In his chapter, Drake provides a critique of the role of voluntary agencies. These organisations acting *for* disabled people are contrasted with those *of* disabled people. The former, largely charity-based agencies, have tended to reinforce a passive, tragic view of disability, one which focuses on individual impairments. Photographic representations are a powerful means of legitimating such images. These agencies have also been influential in confirming the importance of segregated mentalities and the necessity of the goodwill of others through their donations. Drake maintains that support for organisations *of* disabled people is essential in order that discrimination and negative stereotyping are challenged and changed.

The chapter by Fulcher addresses the question of transforming the lives of disabled people. Transformation is seen as involving cultural and economic factors. This basic project raises questions about how we think about policy, practice and their relationship to the task of transformation. Fulcher argues that government policies and ideas tend to distract us from recognising the complexities of cultural and political life. A critique of 'normalisation' is presented, particularly its failure to engage seriously with the material constraints in the lives of disabled people. Three particular projects are identified and three ways of reading them are presented. These include the politics of difference, developing a counter-culture which represents disabled people's art forms, and viewing the disability movement as an example of a new social movement. In conclusion, Fulcher argues, reducing the oppression of disabled people requires the application of materialist sensibilities. This more flexible, dynamic approach to sociological analysis allows for the possibilities of change.

The chapter by Shakespeare examines the questions of identity and imagery, sexual experience, including abuse, and the potential alliance between disabled people and people with AIDS/HIV. By using existing sources and interview data from a group of respondents, Shakespeare explores some key areas of sexual politics in an attempt to develop a social model of sexuality and gender. He contends that questions of power and prejudice, not impairment and physical difference, are central to disabled people's experiences and struggle for positive self and collective identity.

In the final chapter Peters provides some insights into a sociological journey that is both personal and political. Both sociology as a discipline and society at large are depicted as contributing to distorted and negative perceptions of disability. Emerging ideologies – post-modernism, feminism and critical pedagogy – are examined in terms of their potential to create a new discourse on disability identity. This discourse takes the form of a liberation pedagogy that empowers disabled people in ways which enables them to become political advocates. This activity is enhanced as disabled people are able to take pride in this positive self-identity and are able to publicly discuss it.

CHAPTER 8

A critique of the role of the traditional charities

ROBERT F. DRAKE

Power, Norms and 'Normality'

This chapter assesses the challenges to traditional charities posed both by the social model of disability and by the newly emergent Disability Movement. These challenges include a fundamental dispute about the definition of words such as 'normal' and 'disabled'; debate about how disability is to be understood, and arguments over what kinds of actions constitute appropriate or inappropriate responses to disablement.

Norms and the exercise of power

Powerful social groups seek to impose their own values, expectations and beliefs upon society as a whole. Their interests are codified in norms which they aspire to promote to a more general, and ultimately, universal social acceptance. Accordingly, the concept of 'normality', far from describing some natural or preordained state of affairs, instead represents an acknowledgement of the values which have come to dominate in a particular community at any given time. The formation of 'normality' thus results from – and represents – an exercise of power (Gaventa 1980; Lukes 1974; Crenson 1971). Dominant social norms influence the way we act towards individuals and groups. Conformity is rewarded, but those who fail to comply with society's expectations are ascribed with the quality of deviancy (Becker 1963) and are punished, commonly through sanctions applied in a process that Goffman (1964) has termed stigmatisation. For Dahrendorf, the creation of social norms and the measurement of individuals against them represents an act of evaluation. He argues that the same activities may be interpreted and judged quite differently in different societies. Accordingly:

The sanctioning of conformity and deviance in this sense means that the ruling groups of society have thrown their power on to the side of the maintenance of norms. Established norms are, in the last analysis, nothing but ruling norms.

(Dahrendorf 1969:111)

Such ideas are, of course, by no means new. Gramsci (1971 [1948–51]) has enunciated the concept of hegemony whereby the values of an elite group stand dominant within a society, and through the construction and imposition of an all-pervasive ethos, an elite maintains its own interests whilst subordinating those of others. Similarly, Lukes (1974:24) has described how such a mechanism may operate. The formulation of norms constitutes, *ipso facto*, an exercise of power. This is because social norms frame the context within which people conduct their lives. Lukes argues that dominant social forces impose parameters which can, to whatever degree, prevent people from 'having grievances by shaping their perceptions, cognitions and preferences so that they accept their role in the existing order of things'. Lukes contends that this acquiescence occurs because they can see or imagine no alternative to their role, or because they see it as natural and unchangeable, or because they value it as divinely ordained and beneficial.

Corbett (1991) argues that the concept of 'normality' within contemporary British culture contains a paradox, in that it engenders fear and mistrust of difference, but at the same time, promotes individuality as a desirable commodity. The pursuit of individuality is therefore conducted through efforts to excel in culturally valued endeavours such as sport, rather than in risking ridicule and opprobrium by public engagement in socially alien activities. For Corbett, adherence to the tried and tested is matched by suppression of the risky and experimental. The reaction to citizens who do not conform to 'normality' is to seek to change them through punitive treatment, rehabilitation or amelioration. So, for example, in a world which values physical prowess, the wheelchair user begins with an immediate disadvantage. Since few disabled people hold positions of power it is difficult for them to change the norms by which they are compared to – and differentiated from – non-disabled people. If they cannot overturn dominant norms, disabled people may respond to the constraints imposed by a culturally produced and socially sanctioned 'normality', either by acquiescence within a subordinate role or by the rejection of the prevailing norms altogether, so risking the sanctions that follow as a result of their 'pathological' behaviour (Barnes 1990).

The medical model of disability

Clearly then, ideas of hegemony may be applied to the understanding of disablement. In advanced western societies the predominant view of disability is one informed overwhelmingly by medicine. From the medical perspective, people are disabled as a result of their individual physiological or cognitive impairments.

Medicine responds by seeking to cure or rehabilitate disabled people. Such processes aim to return them to the 'normal' condition of being able-bodied. Finkelstein has proposed that disabled people are rendered dependent by this approach, which governs all interactions between the helpers and the helped:

The existence of helpers/helped builds into this relationship normative assumptions. 'If they had not lost something, they would not need help' goes the logic, 'and since it is us the representatives of society doing the help, it is society which sets the norms for the problems' solutions'.

(Finkelstein 1980:17)

Barton (1986) has identified the medical profession as a major force in configuring the perceptions of disablement held by non-disabled people, and he argues that its particular influence has been felt both in terms of a society needing to control a deviant section of its population, and in the creation and provision of a particular form of institutional management and legitimation. A more detailed exposition of the history and nature of the medical model is given in Oliver (1990) and in Barnes (1990). The main point for the present discussion is that a high proportion of traditional social welfare orientated voluntary agencies subscribe to the medical understanding of disability (see, for example, Drake 1994:465).

The social model of disability

In recent years, disabled sociologists (Oliver 1990; Abberley 1987; Finkelstein 1981a; De Jong 1979) and other disabled people (Campbell 1992; Hunt 1981) have challenged the medical account and have developed an alternative discourse which elaborates a social model of disability. From this perspective, people are disabled not by their physical or mental impairments, but by the configuration of a society designed by, and for, non-disabled people (Swain *et al.* 1993). Thus Brisenden argues that he and other people with impairments:

. . . are disabled by buildings that are not designed to admit us, and this in turn leads to a whole range of further disablements regarding our education, our chances of gaining employment, our social lives and so on. However this argument is usually rejected, precisely because to accept it involves recognising the extent to which we are not merely unfortunate, but are directly oppressed by a hostile social environment.

(Brisenden 1986:176)

For the social model then, the locus of interest is not the disabled individual, but the oppressive aspects of the social, political and economic environment in which disabled people conduct their lives.

Traditional charities

Traditional charities engage in a wide range of social activities including education, religion, sport, drama, hobbies and entertainment. Here our concern is with those bodies who take some aspect of social welfare as their focus. Almost invariably, these traditional charities enunciate their identities and interests in accordance with medical classifications of specific diseases. Such agencies are generally perceived as altruistic enterprises which have been set up to care for disabled people. Their place in society is all but unimpeachable, and their roots go deep into British social history.

With the Industrial Revolution and the advent of machinery designed to be operated by the able-bodied, disabled people were progressively excluded from the workplace. This left them dependent upon others for their livelihood (Finkelstein 1981b). Initially, the Church and the poorhouse were two principal benefactors. Organised charity became a third. From the Victorian era onwards, philanthropic societies played a major part in the lives of disabled people. At first, charities gave alms and provided shelter to the deserving poor and the crippled (Ditch 1991). But as the welfare state expanded, disabled people gained access to cash benefits under the social security system. The role of charities gradually changed from alms-giving to the development of services which comprised a variety of projects such as day centres, sheltered workshops and residential homes: locations separate from the everyday social world of work and leisure (Barnes 1990; Handy 1988; Brenton 1985).

Throughout the twentieth century, traditional charities have become increasingly powerful. The image of informal, rough and ready, kindhearted volunteering obscures a concomitant reality of formally constituted organisations employing thousands of salaried professional staff characterised by Brandon as:

voluntary society civil servants [who] rapidly get out of touch, for example with life inside the rundown council housing estates and the mental handicap hospitals. As they get more powerful they get more out of touch. Life looks different from the inside of a BMW.

(Brandon 1988:27)

The British voluntary sector enjoys annual revenues measured in thousands of millions of pounds per year. The total income of the top 500 charities in 1992 exceeded £3 billion (Charities Aid Foundation 1993). Some agencies have substantial reserves. For example, in October 1994, the charity Guide Dogs for the Blind commanded assets of about £160 million (*Independent on Sunday*, 16 October 1994, p. 1). Though agencies describe themselves as being voluntary, the term is used to mean not that they operate solely with free labour (though many do use volunteers) but rather, that they are (a) non-governmental, (b) not-for-profit, and (c) concerned with charitable aims and objectives as defined in law. They are led predominantly by non-disabled people (Drake 1994) and have become increasingly closely involved in the kinds of mainstream provision that were once the preserve of statutory social services (Darvill 1985; Le Grand & Robinson 1984; Payne 1984; Leat Smolka & Unell 1981).

The many traditional charities who subscribe to the medical model of disability specify their purposes in relation to one or a family of medically defined conditions. Examples of these sorts of groups include the Multiple Sclerosis Society, the Schizophrenia Fellowship, the Alzheimers Disease Society and the Motor Neurone Disease Association. Since traditional charities conceive of disability as being the consequence of individual impairments, it follows that for them, change (rehabilitation, adaptation or cure) must also be located within the individual.

The general acceptance of this analysis, which also perceives disability as being problematic, legitimises intervention in the form of ameliorative, palliative and consolatory activity. For example, voluntary agencies have recognised that many disabled people are not able to use public transport. Traditional charities explain this inability by referring to disabled people's tangible limitations: it is self evident that wheelchair users are unable to mount the steps to the high, narrow platforms of buses and coaches. The response of many traditional groups has been to seek to compensate some particular section of the population for their exclusion from the ordinary modes of transport. Charities do this by raising money to provide specially adapted minibuses whose use is confined principally to designated groups of disabled people characterised as being in need and deserving of help. These agencies are content to see their benefaction prominently advertised on the exteriors of the vehicles they supply. Through this act of identification, charities draw a distinction between those who use the philanthropic transport they have provided, and other members of society who do not. The fulcrum of the differentiation is the presence or absence of a particular bodily state or impairment. The value of the differentiation lies in the public's preference for the private motor car, omnibus and train rather than the charity minibus, a choice based not solely on the *forms*, but also upon the *social status*, of these modes of transport. Accordingly, the emphasis of groups led by disabled people themselves has been rather different: they have preferred to campaign for the redesign of public service vehicles.

The philosophy and practices of many of the traditional charities have led to criticism of them by disabled people. These criticisms may be collated in five main categories:

1. the ethos and focus of voluntary action;
2. hegemony, governance and the control of resources;
3. structures and practices within voluntary groups;
4. the use of imagery by charities; and finally,
5. the political inertness of the voluntary sector.

The ethos and focus of traditional charities

I have argued that traditional charities conform to prevailing ideas about the helpers/helped relationship between non-disabled and disabled people (Finkelstein 1981b), in which the helpers invariably occupy positions of power and authority within agencies, and the helped stand in circumstances subordinate to these. Pagel (1988) chronicled initiatives through which disabled people started to come together to challenge the 'right' of charities and professional people to control their daily living conditions. This confrontation has brought into stark relief the power which these groups hold over disabled clients.

Acceptance of the medical model leads charities to ascribe 'needs' to disabled individuals. These 'needs' describe and measure the difference between a disabled person and 'normality'. This world view contains the implicit assumption that disabled people's incapacities prevent them from satisfying their (ascribed) 'needs' from their own resources. If disabled people refuse to acknowledge that these 'needs' actually exist, their reluctance may be deemed an integral part of their 'condition', caused either by a lack of insight or a failure to come to terms with their situation, or it may even be interpreted as purposive pathological behaviour – an act of militancy or outright disobedience (Anspach 1979). From this perspective, it naturally follows that voluntary agencies arrogate to themselves the right to govern voluntary action; to determine its aims, and to configure its operations. Bloor (1986) has argued that principally through the use of social orchestration, disabled people find themselves constrained in roles characterised substantially by passivity and powerlessness.

Non-disabled people's sense of ownership of voluntary action is readily observed where traditional charities have sought to define terms such as 'empowerment' or 'consumer participation'. Since definitions have been constructed within the dominant (medical) framework of understanding, traditional charities have used 'empowerment' to mean the overcoming or assuaging of individual incapacities in the everyday lives of disabled people. Clearly, empowerment used in this sense neither means nor entails the transfer of power away from the non-disabled towards disabled people within the authority-bearing structures of the voluntary agencies themselves. Likewise, 'participation' is more often regarded as an invitation to disabled people to contribute to the project work of an organisation rather than occasioning their involvement in its governance (Drake 1992a; Croft & Beresford 1990; Pearson 1990).

Hegemony, governance and the control of resources

A second criticism levelled by disabled people concerns the occupation by traditional charities of roles or 'social spaces' that disabled people require for their own emancipation. Most of the largest, richest, and best known charities are governed by non-disabled people who control what should be included, and what excluded, from the purposes, objectives and work of their enterprises. When government departments wish to consult disabled people they will treat these major charities as prime conduits for such representations. Likewise, charities encourage the public in the view that it is appropriate to give donations for the provision of help to disabled people, and as vast sums accrue to these large agencies, it is they who decide how the money should be spent. Sutherland's (1981) criticism of this state of affairs is stark and uncompromising. He proposes that the traditional charities maintain organisational structures over which users have no control. As a result, large amounts of money intended to be used for their benefit are expended in ways which serve their real needs very poorly. According to Sutherland, charities are diverting resources which disabled people could themselves administer, and to compound matters, although disabled people are the logical choice of persons to run the organisations that supposedly represent their interests, they are deprived of that employment, which is instead given to non-disabled people. Sutherland summarises his view of these circumstances with the question: 'What is that if not exploitation?'

Disabled people also criticise the cosy proximity between the voluntary sector and the state; indeed many charities depend greatly upon central government for secure sources of funding. With the advent of the contract culture, grants have been progressively replaced by contractual arrangements and so agencies have attempted to become increasingly professional in order to bid successfully for contracts to provide services (Anderson 1990; Fielding & Gutch 1989; Gutch 1989; Kunz, Jones & Spencer 1989). Government money for charities is predicated upon charities' readiness to engage in activities such as community development and project work (see for example, Welsh Office 1991). Whilst resources are readily available for the provision of services to impaired individuals, funds are less forthcoming where groups seek to militate for political and social change (Gunn 1989; Dingle 1987).

Furthermore, as a proportion of total charity incomes and turnover, the amount of government funding for the voluntary sector is highly significant (Charities Aid Foundation 1993; Mabbott 1992). Broady (1989) has calculated that in Wales the national and county associations of voluntary agencies receive about 90 per cent of their funding directly from the Welsh Office. For a charity to lose a government grant is a serious business, since it can lead to job losses, erosion of prestige, and ultimately, loss of public support. So even where charities do desire to change direction, they may be held fast within their specialist, segregative, service providing roles. Oliver concludes that the stance of traditional charities constitutes a sort of usurpation – of money, of resources, and ultimately, of voice:

The continued presence and influence of these traditional organisations is now positively harmful both in terms of the images they promote and the scarce resources they use up. The time has now come for them to get out of the way. Disabled people and other oppressed minority groups are now empowering themselves and this process could be far more effective without the dead hand of a hundred years of charity weighing them down.

(Oliver, 1988:10)

The traditional voluntary sector is well established. Consequently, disabled people's own organisations face several problems in their efforts to develop and expand. First, they may find it difficult to attract funding because many providers of grant aid have already reserved their budgets in favour of supporting the larger, well-known voluntary agencies. Secondly, disabled people's organisations may, for ideological reasons, refuse to take on the carapace of charitable beneficence. In so doing, these groups suffer a number of detrimental consequences. For example, they receive none of the tax advantages enjoyed by charities, and their refusal to describe themselves as being 'needy' makes it harder to raise money from the public at large for their organisational and operational costs – for if there are no 'needs', then why should people give? Thirdly, following on from the previous argument, charities attract funds on the basis that they support 'good causes' and 'deserving cases', whereas disabled people's groups have no truck with raising money through the invocation of public pity. Indeed, the actions of the more radical disabled people's groups are much more likely to provoke the anger and resentment of the community than its general approbation.

Structures and practices

Empirical evidence (Drake 1994; Oliver 1990) indicates that disabled people are substantially absent from positions of power in voluntary agencies. In few of the traditional charities do disabled people occupy the majority of seats on the management committees; a very small percentage of paid staff are disabled, and very few disabled people represent their agencies either on public planning bodies or as contacts to the press and media in general. At the same time the small numbers of groups that are led by disabled people themselves tend to fare badly in the scramble for grant aid from statutory authorities and the government. The structures of voluntary agencies and the practices that they pursue accord with the prevailing social norms discussed earlier in this chapter. Furthermore, Beresford and Harding have recorded some resistance to the desire of disabled people for inclusion in the decision making structures of traditional charities:

. . . it was the executive director of a voluntary organisation who said 'if you regard our handicapped (sic) residents as users then my response has to be different, it would be quite unrealistic to involve most of our severely retarded (sic) residents in the management or development of services'.

(Beresford & Harding 1990:7)

Where disabled people are absent from authoritative positions in voluntary agencies, though they may have informal influence, the structures and goals of charities will ultimately be determined through the hierarchical power exercised by the non-disabled members of the management committees and by salaried professional staff. This is important because, as Griffiths (1990:40) has observed, many voluntary organisations are run on what he calls 'classic service model principles'. That is, they provide services for consumers rather than involving them in the management of programmes and projects. Gouldner has gone further in recognising that:

It is certainly no dark secret . . . that agencies and their programs come to be regarded by their staff as valuable *in their own right*, and they seek to survive regardless of the effectiveness with which they solve the community's problems.

(Gouldner 1969:134)

Stanton (1970) has argued that such survival requires nothing more than that a voluntary organisation can satisfy the requirements of its funding body, as distinct from the wishes of its clients. Where they have been published, disabled people's own wishes often differ substantially from the interests of the traditional voluntary sector. (See, for example, the concerns of disabled people highlighted in any issue of *Coalition* magazine produced by the Greater Manchester Coalition of Disabled People). Some traditional agencies are beginning to accept that they ought to promote disabled people into the higher echelons of their organisations. In January 1995 for example, the Royal National Institute for the Deaf for the first time appointed a deaf person as its director. Whilst such actions may be welcome, they cannot of themselves amount to fundamental change of the kind under discussion in this chapter.

Imagery

In their fundraising, some traditional charities commission advertising and publicity which present disabled people as helpless, dependent and pitiable. Hevey (1992), Morris (1991) and Doddington, Jones & Miller (1994) have argued that such images have a deleterious effect upon the way in which disabled people are perceived. Disabled people's groups have objected strongly to these portrayals of disablement. For example, the Greater Manchester Coalition of Disabled People reported that the director of one charity had declared openly that he was not interested in presenting positive images, and that as long as the money rolled in the end justified the means. The agency had run a particularly negative national billboard campaign and had provoked the Coalition to assert that it was 'high time the Disabled People's movement mounted a bill poster campaign portraying these charity parasites for what they are' (Greater Manchester Coalition of Disabled People 1990:21).

With the advent of charitable advertising on television and commercial radio the question of imagery becomes even more sensitive. The concept of charity is emotionally charged. It carries with it social approbation. Volunteers who raise funds for charity; philanthropists who quietly donate large sums of money; and people who do years of unpaid community work, are accorded high public esteem and are sometimes awarded honours such as the MBE. Helping 'those less fortunate' is a valued activity, the roots of which go deep in British culture. The traditional voluntary agencies are able to harness the values that underpin the concept of charity when they broadcast their appeals. A number of assumptions underlie the images used in charitable advertising. First, charities believe that it is acceptable to publicise medical conditions that the majority of their governors, committee members, directors and staff may not have. Secondly, charities contend that these impairments are undesirable; constitute a personal misfortune; give rise to special needs; and place a moral obligation to help upon the public at large. Thirdly, charities assume that people with such incapacities both want and deserve public support. Fourthly, charities believe that they are able to effect some material change in the state ('plight') of the target disabled population. Fifthly, charities assume that such change is generally desirable and is specifically desired by disabled persons. Sixthly, charities assume that they are the bodies best placed to determine how public donations should be used.

Against this background, disabled people have a hard time promoting quite different images and messages which may include, for example, that they are full citizens whose rights are denied them, or that the way in which non-disabled people have built the urban environment excludes many disabled people from public places and social life. Disabled people demand the opportunity to acquire resources through work, rather than receive largesse through public subscription. Many are angered by their portrayal as objects of pity; an image damaging to their dignity and social standing. Oliver (1990) argues further, that some charities use disabled people's impairments as the 'selling point' or 'product' in their businesses: disability is socially created.

Clearly, personal acts of altruism, the charitable impulse, the sympathy of one human being for another is not at issue here. Disabled people act as generously and charitably as non-disabled people, and it is right that the community should value those of its members who, without expecting any reward, help others in difficulty. But the use of the term 'charity' to describe a particular type of organisation has entailed the transference of these human values to those agencies whose endeavours largely meet with the support of a non-disabled public, but whose aims may not of *necessity* coincide with the wishes of the disabled people whom they identify as a client group. One particularly contentious area of debate in recent times has been the role of the traditional charities in the political arena.

Political inertness

Social change is predicated upon political change. This fact alone constrains many traditional charities who might wish to focus upon social change. Indeed, legislation such as the Charities Acts of 1993, 1992 and 1960, and the relevant case law since 1933 (summarised in Sheridan & Keeton 1983:42–7) have precluded charities from party political action altogether, and have placed tight restrictions upon voluntary groups in their ability to take forward even such political activity as may be non-partisan. The Charity Commission (1994) has made it clear that an institution whose stated purpose includes the attainment of a political purpose cannot be a charity. The Commission relies upon legal precedents established in the Courts, which have held that purposes designed to help the interests of a political party, or to seek or oppose changes in the law or in government policy, are not charitable.

Here is the nub of the matter. A challenge to the medical model of disability constitutes a challenge to dominant social norms, values and expectations. Accordingly, such actions are frequently deemed to be political, and through the media of the judiciary, the Charity Commission, and related legislation, successive governments have effectively sealed off this sphere of activity. Charities, in order to continue to hold charitable status, must remain politically inert. Charitable status is important to these agencies because it constitutes a gateway to public donations and governmental funding. At the same time registration as a charity also establishes the *bona fides* of an organisation in the mind of the public.

Even if party political lobbying and political activity in general were lawful, and pursuit of political ends had no impact upon the acquisition of resources, many charities might yet avoid engaging in it because their understanding of disability was itself non-political. Approaches that concentrate upon altering the personal circumstances of individuals are likely to offer precious little scope for engagement in national politics.

Contrary to the stance of the traditional voluntary agencies, groups of disabled people (such as the British Council of Organisations of Disabled People) believe that disability is, and must be pursued as, a political issue, sometimes even to the point of civil disobedience and direct action (Crow 1990). This being so, there emerges at this juncture an evident mismatch between the compass of charitable action and the aspirations of disabled people. Barton therefore concludes that:

One crucial lesson is the importance of connecting the *personal* with the *political* so that what has been seen in mainly *individual* terms, can be viewed as a social predicament and thus a political issue . . . The task is an immense one – of moving from powerlessness and oppression to self and collective actualization.

(Barton 1986:286)

The disability movement

The paradigmatic differences embodied in the medical and social models of disability have led disabled people to question in diverse ways the legitimacy and usefulness of the charities which purport to help them, and to ask where lies the border between altruism and oppression? In recent years, more and more disabled people have rejected traditional charities outright, and have inaugurated their own agencies. The Derbyshire Coalition of Disabled People has argued that its power arose from the collective strength of its members and the justice of their claim for full participation and equality. The key to success was its members' own active involvement in their own affairs:

It will soon be a thing of the past for disabled people to be patted on the head, stared at, looked down on, patronised and talked over the top of. [In our agency] only disabled members can vote because they are sick of able-bodied people deciding FOR them.

.(Derbyshire Coalition of Disabled People 1989:4)

The British Council of Organisations of Disabled People (BCODP) now has well over 100 member groups. These bodies concentrate not upon the provision of segregated and specialised services, but upon lobbying for political change in order to achieve access to areas of social life hitherto closed to them. In a famous phrase that has been subtly adapted by the Disability Rights Movement, their aim is to boldly go where everyone else has gone before.

These new voluntary groups (*of* rather than *for*) disabled people subscribe to the social model of disability and thus clearly define disablement as a product both of contemporary politics and of the design and maintenance of prevailing social institutions, norms, values and beliefs. The locus of change must therefore be social rather than individual. For disabled people to acquire the citizenship already enjoyed by others, anti-discrimination legislation is needed to enshrine and protect their rights (Barnes 1991). Roger Berry's Civil Rights (Disabled Persons) Bill (HMSO 1994) is the most recent example of a comprehensive attempt to eradicate the disabling propensities of contemporary political, social and economic practices.

The response of the traditional charitable sector

It is still too early to give a definitive account of how traditional charities are responding to the pressures upon them, but a variety of reactions are indicated. Some agencies have either failed to recognise, or have sought to ignore, the changes that are happening around them, and either do not think about how they perceive disability, or see no reason to abandon their focus upon the impaired individual. For example, abiding by what Hevey (1993) calls the personal tragedy approach, the Multiple Sclerosis Society has described itself as offering 'a hope in hell'. Some supporters of traditional charity are actively hostile towards the stance of the disability movement, dismissing its aims as ill-conceived, unrepresentative or simply wrong-headed. Amongst the most visible of these antagonists are the Conservative MPs, James Clappison, Edward Leigh, Richard Spring, Michael Stern and Lady Olga Maitland, whose amendments helped to defeat the Civil Rights (Disabled Persons) Bill. (It later came to light that some of the amendments had been drafted by Parliamentary Counsel on the instructions of the Department run by Nicholas Scott, the then Minister for Disabled People. For the complete record of the report stage debate see Hansard [Great Britain, House of Commons, 6th May 1994: cols 960–1017]).

A less negative but still limited response is found in charities who aspire to subsume or contain 'consumer participation' as just another piece of project work, or a new type of advocacy. Users are offered greater involvement and authority within certain 'compartments' of an agency's work away from the main decision-making structures (Drake & Owens 1992). This kind of reaction allows agencies to avoid fundamental shifts in the existing balance of power.

Other groups, in framing their purposes, accept that they cannot reasonably claim to represent or speak on behalf of disabled people and instead base their legitimacy upon accentuating the needs of parents or carers, or stressing the need for research into the causes of impairment, or by promoting activities concerned with the dissemination of advice and information. In my own research (Drake 1992b) several interviewees from different parts of the voluntary sector indicated these kinds of objectives. One, from an agency whose title and history indicated service to elderly disabled people, when asked to nominate the consumer of his group's services said that 'the constitution clearly identifies it as other groups, other agencies, community and voluntary based organisations'. A second interviewee, from a group concerned ostensibly with physically disabled people, saw 'branches as consumers really'. The problem persists for disabled people, that such agencies remain fixed in the minds of the community as being the main charities concerned with the variety of specific medical conditions. They enjoy substantial media attention and the lion's share of public support. As a consequence, disabled people's own groups remain overshadowed and underfunded.

Welfare pluralism and the pre-eminence of the market-place in contemporary social policy has made another option available to the traditional charities, namely that they be transmuted into professional, mainstream service providers under contract to the state. Notwithstanding the voluntary sector's rhetoric about retaining its independence, many agencies welcomed these opportunities almost from the outset (Payne 1984; National Council for Voluntary Organisations 1980; Northern Ireland Council for Voluntary Action 1987).

A few groups, such as MIND, have acknowledged that much of the criticism voiced by disabled people is valid and these agencies are therefore trying to promote users into key positions in management and planning. Others, like the Spastics Society, have recognised the potency and undesirability of disabling images and have changed their names (the Spastics Society is now called Scope). These groups have begun to promote positive messages about disabled people, but their focus remains personal rather than social, and it is not yet clear whether the changes are deep rooted and profound, or simply stylistic and cosmetic. The empowerment of disabled people requires that those who currently have power must relinquish it, and it is this that the traditional charities find most difficult of all. Even positively orientated agencies find it easier to support broad campaigns for civil rights for disabled people than achieve internal change.

Conclusions

Sociological issues

Until recently, sociological interest has been confined to the understanding of disability as a particular sub-division within the study of deviancy. The analysis at the heart of this paper indicates that sociology must take on new approaches to disablement. Hitherto, disabled people have been treated as little more than subjects for investigation, and social researchers have been content to conduct their enquiries within the framework of understanding provided by the medical model of disability (see, as an example, Miller & Gwynne (1972) and the critique by Hunt (1982)). The aim of such research has been primarily to identify 'the problems of the disabled' and to suggest interventions at the individual level designed to ameliorate or palliate these problems.

However, sociologists working with the social model of disability instead turn their gaze towards the institutions and professions whose influence and activities impinge upon the lives of disabled people. From this starting point, disability arises from a socially created denial of citizenship, and the need for research is manifest at the social and political, rather than individual level. Sociology must therefore look afresh at the social construction of 'normality' and give equal weight to counter hegemonies advanced by disabled people in answer to the medical model. Likewise, traditional research into charities has concentrated hitherto upon social policy issues (Brenton 1985) and organisational structures (Handy 1988; Houghton & Allen 1990) rather than the part played by such agencies in the embodiment and imposition of dominant social norms. What is needed is further sociological investigation of charity as a social institution. At first sight, there is a close relationship between organised altruism and the creation of dependency.

But beyond a shift in the focus of sociological research, Oliver (1992) has called for changes in the governance of the research act itself. Within the social relations of traditional research production, considerable power lies in the hands of the researcher both to define the problem under scrutiny and to interpret the subsequent findings. In such relationships it is difficult for disabled people – as subjects – to counteract (or even to know) the predefined agenda which superintends the investigation. Writers who agree with Oliver (for example, Barton 1994 and Barnes 1991) describe an alternative, emancipatory methodology in which disabled people themselves have genuine control at all stages of the process, with the result that they acquire a means of empowerment rather than experience the reinforcement of their subordination.

What future is there for the traditional charities?

In the light of the critique set out in this paper, and broader criticisms articulated by disabled people at large, it is necessary to ask whether any legitimate role remains for those charities still grounded in the 'individual impairment' view of disability. An acceptance of the social model would entail fundamental changes in their foci, objectives, structures, status and practices. Within such a paradigm, charities would aim to militate for deep and wide-ranging alterations in the fabric and structure of social life: they would have to become *political*.

The charities who are unwilling to change are already, for several reasons, anachronistic. First, the notion of charitable benefaction is anathema to disabled people, and they are rejecting those agencies who espouse it. Secondly, the predominance of the medical model is being placed under increasing challenge by the social model of disability. Since the medical model informs the ethos of traditional charities, they are likely to continue to engage in projects and programmes of action aimed at effecting personal, rather than social change. Thirdly, the apolitical stance of the traditional voluntary sector places it at odds with disabled people's own concerns about citizenship and participation. Fourthly, disabled people are substantially excluded from positions of authority and power within traditional charities and these agencies may therefore be highly unrepresentative of those whom they claim to serve (Drake 1994). If these circumstances remain unaltered, such agencies will continue to lose the support of disabled people who are instead finding their own voice and founding their own groups.

The momentum that built up in support of the ill-fated Civil Rights (Disabled Persons) Bill was indicative of the possibility (or even the probability) of future changes in the prevailing norms and understandings that now define disability. There is a very real prospect that before the end of the century, disabled people will acquire civil rights which will guarantee them equal access to employment, full participation in mainstream education and genuine roles in all areas of public life. As a result, the configuration of the social landscape must necessarily change to extend the rights of citizenship to all, irrespective of their impairments. In these circumstances, those agencies which continue to abide by the medical model (whether as traditional charities or as sub-contractors to the state), will be offering a vision of disability and an approach towards service provision that nobody will need, none will value, and few will buy. It remains to be seen for how long the major funding bodies and the public at large will continue to support these organisations.

This analysis carries far wider ramifications, being equally applicable to social services within the statutory sector. Were disabled people to command incomes and resources through paid work, and were the social and physical environment suitably adapted so as to remove the obstacles that currently deny disabled people their citizenship, what kinds of duties would then remain for the statutory or voluntary services to perform? This question lies outside the scope of the present exegesis, but such conundrums will need to be addressed in future. Whatever may happen in the short term, the ascendancy of a social model of disability holds for disabled people the ultimate prospect that the age of patronage, organised philanthropy and institutionalised charity will finally come to an end.

References

Abberley, P (1987) 'The concept of oppression and the development of a social theory of disability' *Disability, Handicap & Society*, 2(1) pp. 5–19.

Anderson, B. (1990) *Contracts and the Contract Culture*. London: Age Concern.

Anspach, R. (1979) 'From stigma to identity politics' *Social Science and Medicine*, 134 pp. 765–73.

Barnes, C. (1990) *Cabbage Syndrome: The Social Construction of Dependence*. Basingstoke: Falmer.

Barnes, C. (1991) *Disabled People in Britain and Discrimination: A Case for Anti-Discrimination Legislation*. Belper: British Council of Organisations of Disabled People.

Barton, L. (1994) 'Disability, difference and the politics of definition' *Australian Disability Review*, 3: 8–22.

Barton, L. (1986) 'The politics of special educational needs' *Disability, Handicap & Society*, 1(3) pp. 273–90.

Becker, H. (1963) *Outsiders*. New York: The Free Press.

Beresford, P. & Harding, T. (1990) 'involving service users' *NCVO News*, October, pp. 7–8.

Bloor, M. (1986) 'Social control in the therapeutic community: re-examination of a critical case' *Sociology of Health and Illness*, 8:305–24.

Brandon, D. (1988) 'Snouts among the troughs?' *Social Work Today*, 10th November, 27.

Brendon, M. (1985) *The Voluntary Sector in British Social Services*. London: Longman.

Brisenden, S. (1986) 'Independent living and the medical model of disability' *Disability, Handicap & Society*, 1(2) pp. 173–78.

Broady, M. (1989) 'The changing state of the voluntary sector in Wales' *Network Wales*, 66:4–6.

Campbell, J. (1992) *Rights Not Fights*, Speech at the Launch of the South Glamorgan Coalition of Disabled People, Atlantic Wharf, Cardiff, 21st March.

Charities Aid Foundation (1993) *Charity Trends*. Tonbridge: Charities Aid Foundation.

Charity Commission (1994) *Political Activities and Campaigning by Charities*. London: Charity Commission.

Corbett, J. (1991) 'So, who wants to be normal?' *Disability, Handicap & Society*, 6(3) pp. 259–60.

Crenson, M. (1971) *The Un-Politics of Air Pollution*. Baltimore: John Hopkins Press.

Croft, S. & Beresford, P. (1990) *From Paternalism to Participation*. London: Open Services Project.

Crow, L. (1990) *Direct Action and Disabled People: Future Directions*. Manchester: Greater Manchester Coalition of Disabled People.

Dahrendorf, R. (1969) 'On the origin of social inequality', in W. T. Blackstone (ed.) *The Concept of Equality*. Minneapolis: Burgess, pp. 96–114.

Darvill, G. (1985) 'Provision for profit – where does that leave volunteers?' *Involve*, 46 p. 2.

De Jong, G. (1979) *The Movement for Independent Living, Origins, Ideology and Implications for Disability Research*. Michigan: University Centre for International, Rehabilitation.

Derbyshire Coalition of Disabled People (1989) *Heard About?* Chesterfield: Derbyshire Coalition of Disabled People.

Dingle, A. (1987) 'Of their own free will?' *Network Wales*, October, pp. 12–14.

Ditch, J. (1991) 'The undeserving poor: unemployed people then and now', in M. Loney, R. Bocock, J. Clarke, A. Cochrane, P. Graham and M. Wilson (eds) *The State or the Market*. London: Sage.

Doddington, K., Jones, R. & Miller, B. (1994) 'Are attitudes to people with learning disabilities negatively influenced by charity advertising?: an experimental analysis' *Disability & Society*, 9(2) pp. 207–22.

Drake, R. F. (1994) 'The exclusion of disabled people from positions of power in British voluntary organisations' *Disability & Society* 9(4):463–82.

Drake, R. F. (1992a) 'Consumer participation; the voluntary sector and the concept of power' *Disability, Handicap & Society*, 7(3):301–12.

Drake, R. F. (1992b) *'A Little Brief Authority?' A Sociological Analysis of Consumer Participation in Voluntary Agencies in Wales*, University of Cardiff, Ph.D. Thesis.

Drake, R. F. & Owens, D. J. (1992) 'Consumer involvement and the voluntary sector in Wales: breakthrough or bandwagon?' *Critical Social Policy*, 33 pp. 76–86.

Fielding, N. & Gutch, R. (1989) *Contracting In or Out?: The Legal Context*. London: National Council of Voluntary Organisations.

Finkelstein, V. (1980) *Attitudes and Disabled People: Issues for Discussion*. London: Royal Association for Disability and Rehabilitation (RADAR).

Finkelstein, V. (1981a) 'To deny or not to deny disability' in A. Brechin, P. Liddiard & J. Swain (eds) *Handicap in a Social World*. London: Hodder & Stoughton, pp. 34–6.

Finkelstein, V. (1981b) 'Disability and the helper/helped relationship. an historical view' in A. Brechin, P. Liddiard & J. Swain (eds) *Handicap in a Social World*. London: Hodder & Stoughton, pp. 58–64.

Gaventa, J. (1980) *Power and Powerlessness: Rebellion and Quiescence in an Appalachian Valley*. Oxford: Clarendon.

Goffman, E. (1964) *Stigma: Notes on the Management of Spoiled Identity*. New Jersey: Prentice-Hall.

Gouldner, A. (1969) 'The secrets of organizations' in R. Kramer & H. Specht (eds) *Readings in Community Organization Practice*. New Jersey: Prentice-Hall, pp. 132–42.

Gramsci, A. (1971 [1948–1951]) *Selections from the Prison Notebooks*. London: Lawrence & Wishart.

Great Britain, House of Commons (1994) *Parliamentary Debates (Hansard)*, Vol. 242 No. 98, Friday, 6th May. London: HMSO.

Greater Manchester Coalition of Disabled People (1990) 'National campaign fund', *Annual Report 1989–1990*, pp. 12–13. Manchester: Greater Manchester Coalition of Disabled People.

Griffiths, H. (1990) 'Community resource development: a strategy for the 1990s', *Policy Studies*, 11(3):pp. 30–41.

Gunn, L. (1989) 'Planning for change', paper from *Planning for Change*, Social Work Services Group Conference, Edinburgh.

Gutch, R. (1989) *The Contract Culture: The Challenge for Voluntary Organisations*. London: National Council of Voluntary Organisations.

Handy, C. (1988) *Understanding Voluntary Organisations*. London: Penguin.

Hevey, D. (1993) 'The tragedy principle: strategies for change in the representation of disabled people' in J. Swain, V. Finkelstein, S. French & M. Oliver (eds) *Disabling Barriers, Enabling Environments*. London: Sage, pp. 116–21.

Hevey, D. (1992) *The Creatures Time Forgot: Photography and Disability Imagery*. London: Routledge.

HMSO (1994) *Civil Rights (Disabled Persons) Bill, [Bill 91]*. London: HMSO.

Houghton, P. & Allen, G. (1990) *The Fifth Estate*. Birmingham: European Society of Associations Executive.

Hunt, P. (1981) 'Settling accounts with the parasite people: a critique of "A Life Apart" by Miller and Gwynne' *Disability Challenge* 1:38, May.

Kunz, C., Jones, R. & Spencer, K. (1989) *Bidding for Change?* Birmingham: The Birmingham Settlement.

Leat, D., Smolka, G. & Unell, J. (1981) *Voluntary and Statutory Collaboration: Rhetoric or Reality*. London: Bedford Square Press.

Le Grand, J. & Robinson, R. (eds) (1984) *Privatisation and the Welfare State*. London: Allen & Unwin.

Lukes, S. (1974) *Power: A Radical View*. London: Macmillan.

Mabbott, J. (1992) *Local Authority Funding for Voluntary Organisations*. London: National Council of Voluntary Organisations.

Miller, E. J. & Gwynne, G. V. (1972) *A Life Apart*. London: Tavistock.

Morris, J. (1991) *Pride Against Prejudice: Transforming Attitudes to Disability*. London: The Womens Press.

NICVA (1987) *Reaching for the End of the Rainbow*. Belfast: Northern Ireland Council for Voluntary Action.

NCVO (1980) *Beyond the Welfare State?* London: National Council for Voluntary Organisations.

Oliver, M. (1990) *The Politics of Disablement*. London: Macmillan.

Oliver, M. (1988) 'No Place for the Voluntaries' *Social Work Today*, 24th November, p. 10.

Pagel, N. (1988) *On Our Own Behalf*. Manchester: Greater Manchester Coalition of Disabled People.

Payne, J. (1984) *Making Partnerships Work: A Case Study of the Implementation of a Joint Funding Pilot Partnership Policy*, [Working Paper 34]. Bristol: School of Advanced Urban Studies.

Pearson, N. (1990) *Putting People First: Consumer Consultation and Community Care*. Cardiff: Welsh Consumer Council.

Sheridan, L. & Keeton, G. (1983) *The Modern Law of Charities*. Cardiff: University College Cardiff Press.

Stanton, E. (1970) *Clients Come Last*. California: Sage.

Sutherland, A. (1981) *Disabled We Stand*. London: Souvenir Press.

Swain, J., Finkelstein, V., French, S. & Oliver, M. (eds) (1993) *Disabling Barriers, Enabling Environments*. London: Sage.

Welsh Office (1991) *Welsh Office Funding of the Voluntary Sector: A Strategic Statement*. Cardiff: Welsh Office.

CHAPTER 9

Beyond normalisation but not Utopia

GILLIAN FULCHER

This chapter has a realist edge to it: a slightly unfashionable position in this allegedly post-modern era. This means that its view of transformative possibilities is less than Utopian. It is about what is possible, rather than the ideal, and what the possibilities are which a complex analysis suggests they might be. Its realism does not mean it is atheoretical or apolitical. Nor is it the same as naturalism. Realism varies in method and intent (Williams 1980), and it is here that we locate its political possibilities.

The chapter's order is as follows. I discuss the project of normalisation, then briefly describe three small projects with disabled people. Next I consider three readings of a project of beyond normalisation, interrogating the projects via the three readings so as to examine their contribution (limits and possibilities) to the broader project. The underlying questions are: Do these small projects, thus interrogated, reframe the way we ought to think about the ideas of policy, practice, implementation and so on? Hence: What do they contribute to a social theory of disability? What is their relevance to the project of diminishing the oppression of disabled people?

The project of normalisation

The project of normalisation began in the 1960s, in what we call the social services, in Scandinavia, out of concerns for the lives of people with learning difficulties (mental handicap was the term then). Nirje (1985) offers a brief history. Wolfensberger (1983), who is at the University of Syracuse in the US, proffers another, arguing that the term be replaced by that of 'social role valorisation', while Oliver (1994) provides a different reading. Whatever it's called, the project's central principle is 'the creation, support, and defence of *valued social roles* for people who are at risk of social devaluation' (Wolfensberger 1983:234). Both the Scandinavian and, even more so, the American model (Brown 1994:123) rested on assertions about the rights of disabled people. The idea of normalisation has been extremely influential in the modern West in a range of services, but the extent to which such services have been able to enact these rights in areas central to the experience of disabled people has been increasingly questioned in the last decade. Brown (1994) notes some progress but the analysis of the regulation of sexual behaviour of people with learning disabilities 'turns on its head the normalization model of homogenous and consensual values *and* testifies to the power of one interest group to define values at any given point in history' (Brown 1994:135).

While the normalisation project appeared to be radical, its assumptions were functionalist and its ideas and concerns interactionist (Chappell 1993; Oliver 1994). Such a project left untouched fundamental practices such as the professional control of services (Oliver 1994). Thus despite its apparent radicalism, the normalisation project could be relatively easily inserted into policy statements and practices.

Normalisation is claimed as a theory – certainly it is an idea which informs practice – a theory whose limitations Chappell describes firstly, as failing 'to provide a theory of *disability* which takes account of the material constraints in the lives of people with learning difficulties'; secondly, as 'dominated by empiricism and the priorities of professionals'; thirdly, as functionalist 'in its assumptions about the relationship between professionals and disabled people'; and fourthly, as 'idealist both in its adoption of interactionist concerns with deviance, labelling and stigma and its emphasis on attitudes and values' (Chappell 1992:39). With these points we must agree. But Chappell also suggests that 'normalisation fails to locate the experience of people with learning difficulties within a political framework' (Chappell 1992:40). Against that view, I would argue that functionalist assumptions about the social (what we used to call 'the social'), like all other social theories, have political implications: the problem is that the political strategies which derive from a functionalist framework are oppressive to all but the dominant class. But the key point in Chappell's discussion for this paper is the failure of normalisation as a social theory to take account of the material constraints in the lives of disabled people. Which materialist social theory can we draw on? Milner (1993:6ff) distinguishes between rigorous materialism (utilitarianism), weaker versions (Marxism, in its critique of political economy, where culture is secondary), and cultural materialism.

Oliver (1994) provides a materialist critique of the normalisation principle, placing it within a Marxist view of political economy, thereby distinguishing it from other readings of political economy. What is meant by political economy is crucial (Oliver 1994:5). He cites a generally agreed definition of political economy

The study of the interrelationships between the polity, economy and society, or more specifically, the reciprocal influences among government . . . the economy, social classes, state and, status groups. The central problem of the political economy perspective is the manner in which the economy and polity interact in a relationship of reciprocal causation affecting the distribution of social goods

(Estes *et al.* 1982, cited in Oliver 1994:5)

He notes that this definition 'can be incorporated into a pluralist vision of society as a consensus emerging out of the interests of various groups and social forces' (Oliver 1994:3). Thus not all political economy readings of the experience of disabled people contribute to a project of diminishing oppression. Oliver cites Albrecht's account of disability as an instance, noting that it is difficult to disagree with Albrecht's description of how disability is produced in capitalist America but that:

the problem with this pluralist version of political economy is that the structure of capitalist America itself goes unexamined as does the crucial role that the capitalist economy lays in shaping the experience of groups and individuals.

(Oliver 1994:6)

He continues, ·

Exactly the same criticism can be levelled at normalisation theory. Devaluation according to normalisation theory is a universal cognitive process and economic and social conditions are only relevant to who gets devalued.

(Oliver 1994:6)

Thus Oliver argues both that 'inegalitarian social structures cannot be explained by reference only to valued and devalued social roles' and that 'Normalisation can also never serve to transform people's lives' (Oliver 1994:13). While Nirje (1985:66–7) includes normal economic conditions as one of the 'eight descriptive facets' which comprise the normalisation principle, this descriptive inclusion (a wish list?) does not transform the functionalist framework underpinning the normalisation project. A key problem with normalisation theory is that it:

offers disabled people the opportunity to be given valued social roles in an unequal society which values some roles more than others. Materialist social theory offers disabled people the opportunity to transform their own lives and in so doing to transform the society in which they live into one in which all roles are valued.

(Oliver 1994:28)

Beyond normalisation?

The project of transforming the lives of disabled people raises issues which include the theoretical-political matter of how this transformation is to occur. This chapter explores the question of whether transformation can occur with the help of ideas which retain a materialist sensibility but which do not regard cultural practices as secondary to the 'economy'.

What do we mean by the idea of transformation? The term appears in various readings of social life (Foucault 1991:53–9; Oliver 1994:22; Roman 1993a; 1993b), and is generally undefined. But each usage carries a meaning which is to be found within the wider understanding of social life in which it appears. Thus Foucault frequently refers to the idea of transformation (1991:55–9, 70–1), does not define it but emphasises his concern to move from notions of social change, for these imply a change in type or form.

Foucault's work involves an attempt to move beyond dualistic ideas where meanings are, in part, defined by their opposite: luck/planning, change/status quo, normal/abnormal, Gemeinschaft/Gesellschaft. This is because dualistic readings of the social construct misleading questions and analyses. Thus the notion of social change, like other dualisms, is known only by its opposite: as not the status quo (as if that were static). In attempting to move outside such categories, it is useful to read social life as constituted by a complex array of social practices, each of which contains many practices: linguistic and discursive (by which I mean both linguistic and other bodily practices), including deploying phenomena more obviously external to us (as is language in an important sense), such as technology and what we call the natural world. In this context, the idea of transformation is a useful metaphor: it involves an alteration in the strands which interweave to constitute complex social practices, where alterations in what is being transmitted may affect what is happening, or shape outcomes.

An important question underlying this analysis is: What might these small projects tell us about the politics and theory of this task of transformation? Alongside this question, I have two other main concerns. The first concerns our general understanding of, and orientation to, government-level policy for disabled people, or more particularly, how we think about government and the kind of ideas it offers us for thinking about the way we are governed. The dominant ideas it proffers are the themes of policy, practice, implementation, objectives, and, at present, efficiency and effectiveness. Are these useful ideas for gauging differences in disabled people's lives which are claimed to derive from policy 'initiatives'? I have argued elsewhere that they are not. I shall also put aside ideas of progress (an Enlightenment idea), and those of the success and failure (ideas from the achieving society) of policy, for these are peculiar though popular ideas.

Secondly, I want to move from critique (this is relatively easy if you like writing) to a position which some, such as the feminist Leslie Roman (1993), call critically transformative realism: this view about the *political* necessity of realism draws on the work of Raymond Williams, as he put it in his essay 'A Defence of Realism'; 'Any analysis, however academic and theoretical, is put to the hardest test of practice . . . (when) you have to find it somewhere on the ground' (cited in Roman 1993:18). Moreover, 'What is at stake (is) struggles over knowledge claims and representations of "the real" ' (Roman 1993a:22). Taking our critique to what's 'on the ground' might be called a practical bent: but all practice is theorised – thought about – in one way or another. Again, we meet the dualisms in our language and its logic: practice *or* theory? They are not separate. It is for this reason that non-dualistic concepts and analysis are theoretically politically important. Now to the projects.

An arts project

In this project some 200 severely disabled people come each week to create their individual paintings, about twelve people each morning and afternoon. To be accepted as an artist in this project one has to have an interest in, and a capacity to, paint or draw.

Most of the artists do not speak. They work alongside a few highly experienced arts workers whose task it is to provide three kinds of space: the physical space (an easel/table, paints/crayons, etc), the psychological space (a calm environment), and the 'imaginal space' in which the artists are free to create. The arts workers' intervention is minimal: they use speech briefly, to encourage or proffer (What about this colour? Do you think you are finished?).

How the arts workers and painters communicate is largely undescribed: a topic of intense interest and questioning among the arts workers. Between the artist and her canvas there is also, typically, a great deal of communication: some would say that the artist is exploring her sense of herself as separate, and as producer (I have created something outside myself.) One of the artists has paintings hung in European cities, and talks of selling her work. The project regularly holds exhibitions in its own gallery and elsewhere. How the paintings are hung and received is a matter of some concern to the project workers.

Six of the 200 artists receive Federal Government monies under the Supported Employment Scheme: commercial success is being encouraged as well as economic independence. This project receives the Federal Government monies as a community-based programme which is described – in *policy* terms – as providing services in the areas of continuing education, recreation, pre-vocational training, and personal and social development. We can note the rather narrow dimensions of this policy frame.

An undertaking with computers and children diagnosed as autistic

This small project involves computers, children diagnosed as autistic, and a social anthropologist, Roger Coldwell, who has worked on this project intermittently for 20 years. On the one hand, his concern is with individual competence: with the ability of these children to communicate with parents, teacher, carers, by using computers and graphics software. This concern with individual competence is, at one level, within what we might call normalisation, although not closely enough for some of Coldwell's critics who oppose this work as detracting from (normal) 'socialisation' (Coldwell 1993b:1). But as Coldwell (1993a:1) notes, symbols have been central to human means of communication, and symbolic systems have included the Chinese picture system and the Egyptian system of hieroglyphics.

   Coldwell (1993a:3) asks too whether 'our symbolic systems . . . are a major limitation on autistic people communicating effectively', and suggests 'we may be underestimating the potential of some autistic children . . . they seem to have strengths that we are not aware of' (Coldwell 1991a:88). Further, 'with exposure to a graphical system, they did (six children), in fact, acquire skill in using the system that other people denied that they would' (Coldwell, personal communication):

The autistic children would not (perhaps could not) use any of our symbols, whether those symbols are alphabetical, numerical or graphical. I tried getting them to use a set of *Compix* pre-made, drawings of cats, dogs etc. but, no, they couldn't use them. When they drew their own versions, however, they had no problem. Indeed, they were even able to interpret the meanings of one another's symbols.

(Coldwell, personal communication).

Moreover, when he altered one of the children's drawings another would correct it to its original form. This suggests:

[t]here is a . . . characteristic spatial relationship between, and a distinct order to, their symbols. Using fifth generation computer software, we are exploring the possibility of a computer interpreting and responding to relationships and meanings attributed to their symbols. This poses a possibility of their holding a dialogue with a computer and, with the networking of microcomputers, the possibility of their communicating with one another and, given our sympathy, the possibility of their communicating with us.

(Coldwell 1993a:5).

Coldwell (1991b:12) suggests that these children are a 'legitimate sub-cultural group with an ability to develop their own complex communication system' and he (1993a:3) asks whether 'they (can), too, develop their own language' (Coldwell 1993a:3).

Overall, this project goes well beyond a focus on individual competence in communication and on normalisation. In this, it takes issue with a narrow professionalism encouraged by government-level national policy which both in higher education policy (Coldwell works in a university) and in disability policy encourage a managerial, hierarchical professionalism. It raises questions about a language which children diagnosed as autistic may have, how that may differ from the dominant language, and what their means of communication with one another is, as well as the sub-cultural possibilities which may emerge from this work.

People with sight loss: a peer workers project

This project began formally[1] in late 1990, in a large traditional, agency for people with various kinds and degrees of sight loss, where national policy at government level created conditions for practices concerned with, among other themes, 'consumer outcomes' for disabled people. Such ideas can be deployed either to oppress or to diminish that oppression (Fulcher 1992). The project's objective, formulated by a welfare worker and a researcher, was to explore the possibilities of people with sight loss setting up their own service in a Low Vision Clinic where they might be neither clients, patients, volunteers, peer counsellors, aides to the professional staff nor consumers.

The space for this exploration was won by deploying both the notion of consumer outcomes in Federal Government policy, and the (positivist) idea that research (this was a research process initially) was 'technical'[2] and needed 'space'. This was the first contest won and the Steering Committee set up to oversee the process dissolved.

Eight people with sight loss, a welfare worker and researcher met weekly for some 12 weeks. To this exploration the employees brought only (as far as they could be reflective/conscious about themselves) a rejection of the notion of compliance (favoured in the American literature on Peer Volunteers), and a wish to hear the voice of these people. The group appointed a scribe (the researcher) to record the points discussed, resolved and unresolved: these were not minutes, nor was the summary report a training manual. The language was that of the peer workers, the issues covered those of structural differences and personal experience.

Some weeks later, in January 1991, a room was found and the peer workers began work, making themselves available to other people with sight loss who were newcomers to the clinic. Some six months later, the peer workers and the two employees were able to report that staff generally welcomed the 'service', that it was being used, and that an optometrist had reported that 'The peer workers have transformed our work. We can now get on with the technical work because newcomers to the clinic have already talked to someone living with sight loss.'

Since the emergence of peer workers, the agency has cut staff, the researcher has gone, the welfare worker has retired, and the work peer workers do has expanded in kind. They have replaced two paid employees in the technical aids centre, and, as well as the original peer work, they now provide an 'information' service for people who want to know what might lie in store for them when they become 'clients' or 'consumers' at the Clinic. As well, a variety of self-help groups have emerged at various sites in the agency which has offices and facilities throughout the Australian State of Victoria, an area larger than England with a population of around five million. These self-help groups include meetings of a University of the Third Age which non-disabled people also attend. The numbers of peer workers have increased (the service at the original clinic is fully staffed and there are stand-bys) and, in addition to their day-to-day work with newcomers receiving Clinic services, they now also work at four Day Centres. A further effect is that the Blind Members (the legally blind) on the agency Board are more active than were their counterparts or they in 1990.

These effects have not occurred without contention. When the welfare officer retired, an administrator set up a 'training programme' for the peer workers who went along but decided that they didn't need it. An administrator asked whether the peer workers had too much power. The language or discourse of work and of equality – and its associated practices – is constantly contending with a discourse of professionalism where that is deployed as subjugation: to challenge the power of the disabled.

Summary

These are the bare details of the small projects. Even from this brief sketch, it is clear that they raise a number of common issues. These are the importance of means of communication for disabled people other than the dominant focus on individual competence in speech and writing; the struggle over means of communication (see also Fulcher 1992a), against that dominant mode, either in form (speech and writing) or in content (as in the peer workers contending against the kind of roles derived from a particular language about disability which, typically, management would welcome them have); how disabled people are, and how disability is, represented; the much broader issue of the language of disabled people than means of communication. For instance, what is the language which enables severely disabled people and, say, arts workers to communicate so well? What is the nature of the symbolic code which some children diagnosed as autistic appear to have?

Given the commonalities between the small projects, do they contribute to a broader project of beyond normalisation? But first, what might such a project look like?

Materialist sensibilities and the project of beyond normalisation

In this section, I shall discuss three readings of how to reduce the oppression (or marginalisation, which is the concern in the first reading) of disabled people. Each has materialist sensibilities, while not presupposing a clear distinction between materialist and other constraints. The first two accounts are provocative, but I shall argue that a third reading points to the complexities, limits and possibilities of such a project.

Culturally productive action as materialist: claiming difference as legitimate

This reading comes from two Australian academics, Roger Trowbridge and Kate Driscoll, who locate the exclusion (marginalisation is their term) of disabled people both in the economic relations of a global economy and in mainstream culture. In this view, a key to transforming or, at least, diminishing this marginalisation, lies in overcoming the stereotypes both of what is seen as economically productive activity, and of the identity and capacity of disabled people. Here their strategy, or discursive practice, pivots on a particular idea: in their teaching, writing and activism, Trowbridge and Driscoll borrow Melucci's and Boyce's idea of *culturally productive action*, a term they deploy to shift the thinking of both government and recreation workers (Melucci 1988; Boyce *et al.*; cited in Driscoll and Trowbridge, unpublished:2). To this end, they have also sought to encourage recreation workers to work outside a policy for recreation activities which focuses on individual enjoyment, and on individualistic forms of integration (a day at the Zoo, or a football match). Their work aims to go beyond individualistic forms of practice with disabled people to cultural forms of practice such as collectively produced paintings by severely disabled people (these are described more fully in Fulcher 1992). Through such projects they seek to contend with the idea of productivity as belonging only to the 'economic' sphere.

As part of a critical practice against individualism, Trowbridge and Driscoll have encouraged recreation workers in projects where the means of communication go beyond an emphasis on individual competence in speech, writing and painting, and whose products – such as paintings, theatre, etc – assert the legitimacy of disabled people as different. While the small projects Trowbridge and Driscoll have worked on have not been extensively 'evaluated', it is clear from preliminary research and discussion that severely disabled people have gained much from them, and that this work has raised questions in the minds of others such as recreation workers, agency managers and policy makers about the capacities and identities of severely disabled people (Fulcher 1992a).

Theirs is thus a politics of difference. While the politics of difference, and its exclusionary logic, is central in educational apparatuses in the modern West (Barton & Tomlinson 1981; Fulcher 1989) and, more broadly, in global politics,[3] Trowbridge and Driscoll's work is part of the emerging body of work in writing and activism with disabled people which offers the idea of difference as one factor in a series of relational developments (Oliver 1992; Branson & Miller 1989; Barton 1994) towards diminishing oppression.

Disability representation and the materiality of culture

In Britain, Simon Hevey (1993) writes about disability representation and the oppression of disabled people. He argues that the idea that thinking about the way disabled people are represented in terms of positive images rather than negative images is neither a cultural nor political advance. Instead, Hevey (1993:429) argues for 'political creativity within and about the disability struggle' where 'a sense of self is related to the artist's 'relationship to the movement'. This involves a series of tactics in which he claims it is only the disability arts movement that has taken the opportunity presented by 'the recent shift in economic and social relations consequent on the new electronics and cybernetics revolution' (Hevey 1993:426).

Hevey (1993) describes the oppression of disabled people as deriving from the economic relations of production, the cultural oppression of disabled people associated with the position of 'the flawed body' in western culture[4] and from the anxieties of the able-bodied about their own position in the labour market. In this view of cultural and psychological processes, the flawed body embodies the anxieties of the able-bodied, and the notion of disability is a hologram constructed by the able-bodied for whom it has cathartic effects. Thus, as do others (Abberley 1987; Fulcher 1989; Shakespeare 1994), Hevey distinguishes between impairment and disability, and also argues for shifts in representation as a crucial tactic in diminishing the oppression of disabled people. He therefore asks:

just what is being represented in general disability representation. What is it that unites practically the entire discourse, from Greek Theatre to James Bond villains to Charity Advertising to all the Richard III's, Ravens . . . and so on? *In a word, it is that disablement means impairment and impairment means social flaw.* Thus, we can say that the basic rule of oppressive disability representation is that it is predicated on the social non-worth of an impairment or the person with an impairment.

(Hevey 1993:424)

The flawed body thus occupies a culturally strategic position as embodying the tragedy principle in the cultural of the modern West.

The *tragedy principle*, then, positions a flaw on the body related to the deepest possible social fall. Where impairment enters, the character is proven to be socially dead . . . Whether in television, theatre, cinema, fine art or charity advertising, the tragedy principle uses the impairment as a metaphor and a symbol for a socially unacceptable person and it is this tragedy principle which is the bone-cage surrounding historical and current disability representation. It is this impairment-as-social-flaw that we mean when we say 'negative' representation and it is this that we have to end. This will be difficult because such readings have become 'natural' within representation.

(Hevey 1993:425–6)

Thus, if we follow Hevey's psychological reading a little further, we might read attempts to replace negative images of disabled people with positive images unreconstructed as a repression of the tragedy principle, rather than a freeing of disabled people from this position.

In opposition to the tragedy principle, the individualistic focus of western high culture makes heroism a central theme (the music of Beethoven, the Sagas, folk tales, etc). Hevey's approach to reducing the oppression of disabled people thus involves developing a counter-culture to the tragedy and heroism in western culture, in part, by moving the focus from the 'flawed' body. Disabled people need to control the meaning of artistic practices by controlling how these practices are positioned: the context in which, for instance, paintings are hung. He calls this a political poetic. But can we control these meanings? You and I may look at the 'same' picture but we may read what that picture represents quite differently.[5] In sum:

The cultural task for disabled artists and culture workers is threefold. First, how to 'reclaim' impairment away from a social flaw. Secondly, how to shift disability representation off from the body and into the interface between people with impairments and socially disabling conditions and, thirdly, how to create aesthetic forms which are seen to deal with this successfully (i.e. which can be internalised by disabled people in struggle.

(Hevey 1993:426)

Hevey argues that it is:

both the organisation of economic production *as well as* the projection of (non-disabled) negative desire, which contains disabled people within oppressive cultural representation.

(1993:426)

Thus 'a shift in the surrounding social relations and economic conditions are also necessary'. The recent shift in economic relations associated with 'the electronics cybernetics revolution' offers opportunities for disabled people. The new activism (in Britain) has emerged, and part of its task in representational terms is 'the *de-biologisation* of the disability', that is, 'shifting the focus *away from the body and onto society*' (p. 427). While the de-biologisation of disability and its urgent recognition both as a construct which government uses to regulate (Fulcher 1989a), and as an object on which the able-bodied can project their negative desire (Hevey 1993), is at one level important, it raises other problems.

Hevey's dualism of the body and society is, in a Foucaldian reading, too simple. We all, not just the disabled, are governed by the coercion and production of docile bodies. This occurs both in the 'economic' and 'cultural' spheres, and more broadly: the social enters into, is constituted, in part, by the regulation of the body. Thus Foucault (1977:151ff), for instance, was interested in 'how deployments of power are directly connected to the body'. It is not just that there are gestures, habits of speech, of ingestion and excretion that are historically and culturally variable as norms: they appear to be socially implanted in the body's mechanisms, beyond levels of consciousness (Freund 1988). It is in this sense, and in others, that society is in the body (see also Freund 1988:544–5; Hewitt 1993).

Hevey also argues that:

The disability arts movement is the first sign of a post-tragedy disability culture. To state this clearly, the disability movement is the articulation that (a) impairment and disability are no longer focused as one, and (b) they are no longer *exclusively* focused on the body. The disability arts movement is the only area which is dealing with the cultural vacuum which now exists given this shift.

Thus Hevey's writing on disability arts is more broadly part of a tradition on the revolutionary potential of art, a tradition which claims culture as not secondary to some more basic phenomenon but as having materialist realities and transformative possibilities. This is to argue, at the very least, that artistic practices with a political poetic (itself a complex idea and practice – not to be identified as necessarily a characteristic of the artistic products of disabled people) raise issues of awareness, consciousness, constituency and therefore political mobilisation.

There are parallels here with feminism, since part of feminist strategy has been to raise consciousness about oppression, and the tactics Hevey advocates, such as positioning the issue on to the issue, resonate with the strategies some aboriginal artists in Australia have adopted as part of a complex response to oppression. The photographic compositions of Leah King-Smith impose nineteenth-century photographs of aboriginals on nineteenth-century photographs of the landscape. In colonial Australian art, the landscape is typically represented as either unpeopled, or as peopled by whites (often with romantic themes of loss, isolation and heroism). King-Smith's compositions represent precisely the issue of the relationship between aboriginals and the land. Moreover, her techniques, including the blurring of outlines through superimposing photographs, project that relationship as it is claimed to be traditionally: as mystical and spiritual (Fulcher unpublished).

Normalising tendencies and cultural materialism

These two readings of how to diminish the oppression (or marginalisation is Trowbridge's and Driscoll's frame) of disabled people do not rest on the notions of abnormal/abnormal. But as Oliver (1994:12) notes, the project of normalisation does. What is the relevance of this duality to our thinking about a project of beyond normalisation?

The ideas of normal and abnormal are problematic, not only morally and politically but epistemologically. Despite traditional dualism having been demolished by seventeenth- and eighteenth-century scientists (Noam Chomsky, ABC Science Show, 18 February 1995), our language is saturated with such concepts: a legacy of Cartesian categories. The drawbacks of analyses based on dualisms has been a topic of sociological discussion for some time. A more complex analysis of social life as constituted by an array of interrelated practices, each with, as it were, constituent elements (it is difficult to avoid essentialism here but that is not what I mean), may provide an analysis which overcomes the black–whiteness of oppositions in Cartesian thought.

The notion of normal and abnormal may be seen as underpinning normalising judgements. Foucault usefully links the idea of normalising judgements with the operation of power through the idea of *normalising tendencies*. This idea overcomes the untheorised oppositions to, or dualisms of, the idea of normalisation and its alternatives, such as liberation. Foucault draws our attention to the *ever present tendency to practices which normalise*. This leads not to the notion of liberation but to the idea of the possibilities of political practices (James 1987:90) in particular arenas: and it intimates too, the idea that there may be *shifts in politics* but that the *struggles remain* (Fulcher 1993).

The notion of tendency points to flexibilities, uncertainties and possibilities, rather than absolutes or clear dichotomies (things are clear and of *this* or *that* sort) which presume we can distinguish between normal and abnormal on the ground. If we move from black and white thinking, we might suggest, in some instances, that the dominant tendencies might lead the dominant class or majority to pronounce in this way: this is an instance of *this* categorical (dualistic) event. If we drop the alleged reality of the dichotomy between normal and abnormal, while still recognising its normative importance, we can see that we are all subject to ever-present normalising tendencies: as men, or as women, with or without impairments, of a certain class, occupation, age, nationality, and so on. But the dominant class has more freedom from these than others (Corbett 1991).

The dominant normalising tendencies in the modern West include the idea that paid work is the prime moral value (Fulcher 1989b): earn, compete as an independent, excluding individual, and value this most highly. A public servant (the funder of the project?) opened an exhibition of paintings by intellectually disabled people in the National Gallery of Victoria, eulogising these ever-present normalising tendencies. Thus she referred not to the nature or content of the art but to 'a belief in the individual's right to compete . . .'; 'the paintings as reflecting the individual perception of the painter . . .'; 'one of the artists competing as a professional is competing in a field of 350'.

If we reject the ideas of normalisation and beyond normalisation and look, instead, at political and cultural life through the idea of ever-present normalising tendencies, we can glimpse limited, temporary and contingent freedoms. These are worth struggling for. Their achievement may be sought not in the slogans of political parties, nor in policy statements, but in analyses of the cultural and political institutions of the modern West. This Foucauldian reading of ideas about normality as constituted by ever-present normalising tendencies can be claimed as having materialist sensibilities. Bennett (cited in Milner 1993:10), for instance, has recently sought to show the materialist position in Foucault's work.

We can combine Foucault's ideas here with Raymond Williams' project, for Williams (1980:87) sought to establish the materiality of culture (Milner 1993:8), arguing that 'whatever purposes cultural practice may serve, its means of production are unarguably material'. Thus Williams coined the term *cultural materialism* to indicate a social theory in which cultural practices were not secondary to the 'economic'. Cultural materialism

is a theory of culture as a (social and material) productive process and of specific practices, of 'arts', as social uses of material means of production (from language as material 'practical consciousness' through to mechanical and electronic communications systems.

(Williams 1980:243, cited in Milner 1993:9)

In his seeking to outline the transformative possibilities within this view of cultural and political life, Milner (1993:59) notes that Williams sought

those particular elements within the more general culture which most actively anticipate subsequent mutations in the general culture itself; . . . (those which) are quite specifically counter-hegemonic.

(Milner 1993:59)

Thus Williams (1977:122) distinguished between *archaic, residual* and *properly emergent cultural elements*. Residual elements may be incorporated into the dominant culture or be in oppositional or alternative relation to that culture: the latter have transformative possibilities. Properly emergent elements need to be distinguished from the merely novel. The former are those 'genuinely new meanings and values, practices, relationships and kinds of relationship, which are substantially alternative or oppositional to the dominant culture' (Williams 1977:123), and it was in this context that Williams saw artistic practices as especially interesting. But emergent elements may also entrench the dominant culture.[6]

What are the political possibilities in Williams' project of cultural materialism? Williams linked these ideas of properly emergent cultural elements with the notion of 'structure of feeling' (1977; 1981), a now problematic idea and in his later work (1989) with the new social movements. Milner (1989:115) suggests that the political possibilities 'seem very much more amenable to alignment with an emancipatory than with an exploitative or oppressive politics'. But he also notes that 'labourisms and radical nationalisms' such as Williams'

> whatever their original emancipatory intent, articulate a by now demonstrably residual, rather than emergent, structure of feeling, in a world that is increasingly internationalised, increasingly post-industrial, increasingly individualised, in short, increasingly 'post modern'.

> (Milner, 1993:115)

Nevertheless, as Milner (1993:57) notes, Williams' earlier words on dominant social orders (1977:121) are worth recalling 'no mode and therefore no dominant social order, and therefore no dominant culture ever in reality includes or exhausts all human practice, human energy, and human intention', as are Milner's on the political possibilities of the new social movements:

> It is, in my view, precisely in the strength both of Williams's endorsement of the new social movements, and of his deliberately nuanced appraisal of the labour movement, that he succeeds in recuperating the positive, but not the negative and fashionably *declassé*, moment within postmodern leftism: 'The real struggle has broadened so much', Williams wrote in *Towards 2000*, 'the decisive issues have so radically changed, that only a new kind of socialist movement, fully contemporary in its ideas and methods, bringing a wide range of needs and interests together in a new definition of the general interest, has any real future' (ibid.:174). This seems to me about as right as we are likely to get it.

> (1993:118)

What does this cultural materialist reading, which draws on both Foucault and Williams, suggest we ask of the three small projects described above?

Interrogating the small projects

Four questions come immediately to mind:

1. What are the ever-present normalising tendencies in these projects?
2. To what extent do they work for the dominant social order and against a project of diminishing the oppression of disabled people?
3. Are there, in these undertakings, the kind of properly emergent cultural elements Raymond Williams describes?
4. Does the analysis suggest we read government policy other than through its ideas of policy and implementation, success and failure?

These are interrelated questions.

In the arts project, the ever-present normalising tendencies include the commercial success required of those in the Supported Employment Scheme, the idea of the commercially successful artist, and the dominant practices which surround that idea and the exclusionary tendency to view this art as that of the Other. In the project with computers, the tendencies are again subtle: for instance, the stress on individual competence, the rejection of this work by other professionals, the assumptions that autism is a clear diagnostic category which involves an incapacity to communicate. In the peer worker project, these tendencies include extracting more from labour (cut costs: unpaid workers are welcome; become a volunteer; the idea of charity); those which emanate from the deployment of a particular kind of professionalism (one of control by some managers: 'I'm not going to be told by the peers what they're going to do'); and the dominant cultural themes of tragedy and heroism as Hevey describes them (impairment, therefore doom). It is against such tendencies (I am old, have lost most of my sight, and am therefore worthless) that peer workers themselves, at least initially, must often struggle. In so doing, they work against this orientation among those around them.

Our second question draws attention to the struggles, dilemmas and contradictions which characterise these sites. The arts project is a site where the arts workers and the project's director struggle against the ever-present normalising tendencies outside that site; not only of the commodification of the artists' work, although in part they might support this (here is a dilemma) but also against those ever-present normalising tendencies which encourage the view that the paintings may be 'primitive' or, at best, the work of 'the Other'. They struggle against exhibiting the art in galleries where either these tendencies or those of charitable condescension may prevail. There is a contradiction for these workers between encouraging severely disabled people to engage artistically with their canvas in a context which simultaneously carries the dilemma which government-level policy (and its funds) bring: that it rewards paid art, or the attempt to move into the category of paid artist, and that such practices continue to exclude those severely disabled artists who, for reasons perhaps unrelated to their work, will never make it. These are the contradictions in a 'program' which is about including disabled people and providing them with equal rights.

In the computer project the psychologist struggles against the controversy this work raises, and the disbelief this entails at many levels. The site in which the peer workers practice contains contradictions at a number of levels: the corporate, professionalised, managerial, hierarchical culture is at odds with a properly equitable solidaristic undertaking with those deemed most in need of 'help'; this produces ongoing contests. Moreover, peer workers aren't paid but are not, as yet, contained as 'volunteers'; but this practice contradicts the politics and morality of paid work which is a dominant cultural element not only in the site, but outside it. Some peer workers have (had) a contradictory subjectivity, at least initially, struggling against the theme – I am old, have lost (some of) my sight, etc. Similarly, as was evident in the 'research' process (the weekly discussions before setting up the service), some future peer workers struggled against further aspects of a contradictory subjectivity. These derived from gender (most were female), the wish to make their voice and experience heard, and years (because these people were mainly 50 and over) of alternate ideas, from an era when the voice of the disabled, and that of women, was hardly heard, in the sense of being listened to. Coincidentally, they struggled against the possibility of losing their voice not to a medical discourse but to another professional discourse, that of sociological terms (structural issues were never proffered as necessary but were arrived at by the peer workers). Thus they carefully weighed the meanings of words and returned to them.[7] Further, the extent to which peer workers retain control of their immediate practices is a continuing struggle in this site, while the key issue for disabled people is the extent to which they gain control of overall services (Oliver 1988; 1989; 1994).

Further, the extent to which these undertakings contribute to a social order which does not exclude disabled people is, at one level, limited. Firstly, insofar as they are unrelated projects, their effect is limited. Moreover, the institution, the agency for people with sight loss, remains and the control disabled people exert over their services is limited, challenged, but increasing. No particular outcome can be guaranteed. Despite their lack of connection with one another politically, as a movement rather than as individual sites governed in part by government policy 'initiatives', these undertakings may, nevertheless, be seen as significant. Gorz (1973) argues that transformation is a cultural task and a matter of small reforms. He sees the 'work of ideological research and formulation, apart from its political aspects, (as) . . . a *cultural* undertaking' (Gorz 1973:170). Further, 'anti-capitalist reform, which is synonymous with revolution . . . has to be brought about by the creation of an anti-capitalist block, by mass struggle for reforms which will set the revolutionary process in motion' (Gorz 1973:52).

In part, our answers to the second and third questions depend on identifying the cultural elements present in these sites. Are they archaic, residual or properly emergent, or do they contain all three? In each, there are practices with cultural elements which mitigate against the ever-present normalising tendencies.

In the arts project, there are subtle, important, and largely unarticulated means of communication between arts workers and artists, between the artist and her canvas, and between these canvases and the people who see them. My reading is that there are largely unarticulated but potentially very emergent cultural elements in this site. Similarly, in the computer project, the possibility of a sub-culture of children diagnosed as autistic has appeared. At the same time, might the emergence of such a sub-culture indicate exclusionary possibilities for other sections of the population? There is now the possibility that various computer languages will become major means of communication, at the same time excluding those who are unfamiliar with, or lack the technology to, communicate in this way over vast or small spaces. Thus there may be both properly emergent cultural elements in this site but emergent defensive elements occurring more broadly. In the agency in which peer workers now work unpaid, as against the ever-present normalising tendencies of charity (subtle undertones remain), and the deployment of a particular kind of professionalism, the 'new voices' and practices of peer workers are also present, and these have increased in the agency in the three years since the project began. To the extent that the discursive practices ('voice' and practice) of the peer workers are different from the kind of peer counsellor projects reported in the American literature, which are largely concerned with compliance, these practices may constitute properly emergent cultural elements.

This analysis of these undertakings and these sites offers a dynamic reading of cultural and political life which avoids the misleading analyses which emerge from the kind of dualisms present in static analysis. In part, in my view, the possibility of new social orders lies in reading the struggle between the dominant ever-present normalising tendencies and properly emergent cultural elements.

On the fourth question, the ideas of contradiction, dilemma and struggle are not part of the discourse of government or its policy analysts, nor are they themes which typically characterise discourse about social policy. Governance in Australia, and more broadly in the modern West, occurs in important respects through a medium of words like 'consensus' and 'participation'. The neat ideas government provides us with to understand how we are governed are inadequate: they distract us from a more complex political reading. The ideas of policy, programme, implementation, objectives, outcomes provide a rational reading of a deeply political reality. The reality is different: it is that of struggles, contradictions and dilemmas. Thus this reading of cultural and political life requires a quite different set of ideas from those that government proffers. To say this is also to support earlier arguments about the irrelevance of the Parliamentary process to reform (Gorz 1973:44; Hindess 1981).

These small undertakings demonstrate the practical, therefore theoretical/political, irrelevance of these terms in understanding how, in this instance of political life, the oppression of disabled people continues to occur, right in the middle of a 'program' which is allegedly about helping disabled people. Such programmes are often welcomed uncritically. On the other hand, we can see that in these sites of struggle, some small freedoms occur which coincidentally work against that oppression.

Conclusion

How do these small freedoms and these superficially unrelated projects contribute more broadly to diminishing the oppression of disabled people?

In part, by requiring us to interrogate our readings – our theorising therefore our politics – of socio-political and cultural life; in part, by the changed experience of disabled people in these sites; also, by encouraging us to reflect about the possibilities of similar critical realist analyses in other projects, and the transformative possibilities not only in them but more broadly, in a social movement of disabled people.

Further, the small undertakings suggest some of the sociological tasks in this project. These include firstly, further exploration of the nature of language whereby severely disabled people and others, such as arts workers, communicate well. Secondly, it suggests we think about the representation which the cultural products of disabled people convey, and the possibilities which Hevey's analysis suggests, as well as the limits of that analysis. Thirdly, it suggests we reframe our examination of government policy. It suggests that sociological questions are different from those of government. Such an analysis discourages reactionary politics, and simple calls for policy reforms. Finally, sociological analysis which notes the fragmentation, and possible articulation, of such small projects within a wider theory of governance and movements around it, may also contribute to reducing the oppression of disabled people.

What this theorising has suggested is the limits and possibilities – the complexities – of a project of beyond normalisation, and of the need, as the feminist Leslie Roman (1993:23) points out, for people, in producing themselves and their situations, to continually evaluate different alternatives and courses of action.[8] In addition, the materialist sensibilities of the cultural analysis offered here, which argues that the task of transformation is as much cultural as 'economic', reveals that the ideas government proffers for thinking about politics and political life, including the idea of 'policy for' disabled people, are a distraction from recognising the complexities of cultural and political life: these include ever-present normalising tendencies, and a range of cultural elements which may or may not work towards new social orders. It is in this sense that a cultural analysis with materialist sensibilities contributes to a social theory of disablement as it is presently constructed.

Notes

1 Earlier it was an idea in the mind of the welfare worker.
2 It never is merely this. It is also political.
3 But specific localities may make a difference. Thus Bouma (1995) argues that the emergence of religious pluralism in Australia is occurring under specific conditions and factors compared with some other societies in the modern West.
4 This is not to sustain the divisions between high and low.
5 On the politics of representation, see Shapiro (1988).
6 See Roman (1993b) on emergent defensive racism.
7 On reflection, the process shared aspects of Leslie Roman's (1993a, 1993b) description of her pedagogical critically transformative realism.
8 See Roman (1993) on Brecht's drama and Williams' unfinished project of a socially transformative critical realism.

References

Abberley, P. (1987) 'The concept of oppression and the development of a social theory of disability' *Disability, Handicap & Society*, (2)1, pp. 5–20.

Barton, L. and Tomlinson, S. (eds) (1981) 'Introduction: a sociological perspective' in Barton, L. and Tomlinson, S. (eds) *Special Education: Policy, Practices and Social Issues*. London: Harper and Row.

Bouma, G. (1995) 'The emergence of religious pluralism in Australia: a multicultural society' *Sociological Analysis*, 56(2), 1995.

Branson, J. and Miller, D. (1989) 'Beyond integration policy – the deconstruction of disability', in Barton, L. (ed.) *Integration: Myth or Reality*. London: The Falmer Press.

Brown, H. (1994) ' "An Ordinary Sexual Life?": a review of the normalisation principle as it applies to the sexual options of people with learning disabilities' *Disability & Society*, 9(2), pp. 123–44.

Chappell, A. L. (1992) 'Towards a sociological critique of the normalisation principle' *Disability, Handicap & Society*, 7(1):35–51.

Coldwell, R. A. (1991a) 'Computers in use by autistic children: some case studies' *Proceedings of the Ninth Australian Computers in Education Conference*, at Bond University, Gold Coast, September:94–100.

Coldwell, R. A. (1991b) 'Intellectually handicapped children: development of hieroglyphic symbols' *Australian Educational Computing*, September:10–12.

Coldwell, R. A. (1993a) 'Development of symbolic systems on computers by autistic children' *Att Undervisa* (published in Swedish) 2, pp. 23–6.

Coldwell, R. A. (1993b) 'Artificially intelligent communication for autistic children' Draft research note on methodology sent to *Att Undervisa* for translation into Swedish, typescript, 3 pp.

Coldwell, R. (1994) personal communication, June 1.

Corbett, J. (1991) 'So, who wants to be normal?' *Disability, Handicap & Society*, 3, pp. 159–60.

Driscoll, K. and Trowbridge, R. (unpublished) 'Disability and Aged care – emergent themes in social policy' Department of Leisure and Tourist, Royal Melbourne Institute of Technology, paper to Australian Social Policy Conference, 1993, typescript, 10 pp.

Finkelstein, V. (1980) *Attitudes and Disabled People – Some Issues for Discussion*. New York: World Rehabilitation Fund.

Foucault, M. (1977) *Discipline and Punish: The Birth of the Prison*. Harmondsworth: Penguin Books.

Foucault, M. (1991) 'Politics and the study of discourse' in Burchell, G., Gordon, C. and Miller, P. *The Foucault Effect: Studies in Governmentality*. London: Harvester Wheatsheaf.

Freund, P. E. (1988) 'Bringing society into the body' *Theory and Society*, 17:839–64.

Fulcher, G. (1989a) *Disabling Policies? A Comparative Approach to Education Policy and Disability*. Lewes: Falmer Press.

Fulcher, G. (1989b) 'Disability: a social construction' in Lupton, G. M. and Najman, J. M. (eds) *Sociology of Health and Illness: Australian Readings*. South Melbourne: Macmillan.

Fulcher, G. (1992a) *Pick Up the Pieces! What do Recreation Workers Need to Know About Working with People with Severe Disabilities?*, Report prepared for the Department of Leisure and Recreation, Phillip Institute of Technology, Bundoora, Victoria, 121 pp.

Fulcher, G. (1992b) 'Pigs' tails and peer workers: the view from Australia' in *Disability: The Necessity for a Socio-Political Perspective* (with Len Barton and Keith Ballard), published by The International Exchange of Experts and Information in Rehabilitation (IEEIR) in association with the University of New Hampshire, monograph #51 in the WRF-IEEIR series.

Fulcher, G. (unpublished) 'Modern identity and severe disability: how might recreation workers encourage people with severe disabilities to live? Towards a framework' paper prepared for the Department of Leisure and Tourism, Royal Melbourne Institute of Technology, Melbourne, Australia, typescript, 91 pp. plus 17 pp. pictorial text, 18 December 1993.

Gorz, A. (1973) *Socialism and Revolution*, Anchor Press edition (trans. by Norman Denny).

Hevey, D. (1993) 'From self-love to the picket line: strategies for change in disability representation', *Disability, Handicap & Society*, 8(4), pp. 423–9.

Hewitt, M. (1993) 'Bio-politics and social policy: Foucault's account of welfare' *Theory, Culture & Society*, 2(1), pp. 67–84.

Hindess, B. (1981) 'Parliamentary democracy and socialist politics' in Prior, M. (ed.) *The Popular and the Political: Essays on socialism in the 1980s*. London: Routledge and Kegan Paul, pp. 29–44.

Hindess, B. (1986) 'Actors and social relations', in Wardell, M. L. and Turner, S. P. (eds) *Sociological Theory in Transition*. Boston, Mass.: Allen and Unwin, pp. 113–26.

James, P. (1987) 'Theory without practice: the work of Anthony Giddens' *Arena*, 78:26–9.

Milner, A. (1991) 'Raymond Williams' in Beilharz, P. (ed.) *Social Theory: A Guide to Central Thinkers*. St Leonards: Allen and Unwin.

Milner, A. (1993) *Cultural Materialism*. Carlton: Melbourne University Press.

Mitchell, R. (1990) 'A liberation model for disability services' *Australian Disability Review*, 3(90), pp. 31–6.

Nirje, B. (1985) 'The basis and logic of the normalization principle' *Australia and New Zealand Journal of Developmental Disabilities*, 11(2), pp. 65–78.

O'Connor, A. (1989) *Raymond Williams: Writing, Culture, Politics*. Oxford: Basil Blackwell.

Oliver, M. (1988) 'Disability and dependency: a creation of industrial societies?' in Barton, L. (ed.) *Disability and Dependency*. London: The Falmer Press, pp. 6–22.

Oliver, M. (1989) 'The social and political context of educational policy: the case of special needs' in Barton, L. (ed.) *The Politics of Special Educational Needs*. London: The Falmer Press, pp. 13–31.

Oliver, M. (1992) 'Intellectual masturbation: a rejoinder to Soder and Booth' *European Journal of Special Needs Education*, 7(1), pp. 20–8.

Oliver, M. (1994) 'Capitalism, disability and ideology: a materialist critique of the normalization principle' typescript, 30 pp. Paper presented at an international conference on normalisation, at the University of Ottowa, Canada.

Pane, L. G. (1993) 'A triple (dis)advantage: women with disabilities from non-english speaking backgrounds' *Australian Disability Review*, (3)93, pp. 57–65.

Roman, L. G. (1993a) 'Raymond Williams's unfinished project: the articulation of a socially transformative critical realism' *Discourse*, 13(2), pp. 18–34.

Roman, L. G. (1993b) ' "On the Ground" with antiracist pedagogy and Raymond Williams's unfinished project to articulate a socially transformative critical realism' in Dworkin, D. L. and Roman, L. G. (eds) *Views Beyond the Border Country: Raymond Williams and Cultural Politics*. London and New York: Routledge.

Shakespeare, T. (1994) 'Cultural representation of disabled people: dustbins for disavowal?' *Disability & Society*, (9)3, pp. 283–99.

Shapiro, M. J. (1988) *The Politics of Representation: Writing Practices in Biography, Photography, and Policy Analysis*. Wisconsin: The University of Wisconsin Press.

Thornton, P. (1993) 'Communications technology – empowerment or disempowerment? *Disability, Handicap & Society*, 8(4), pp. 339–49.

Trowbridge, R. (unpublished) 'Culturally productive action: a response to personal and social marginality' paper presented to the Senate Standing Committee on Community Affairs Seminar: Employment of People with Disabilities, typescript, 4 pp., 2 September 1992.

Trowbridge, R. and Driscoll, K. (unpublished) 'High support needs and the politics of choice' paper for My Day My Choice Conference, Melbourne, typescript, 6 pp., 15 July 1993.

Wickham, G. (unpublished) 'Justice, democracy and the demise of politics', typescript, 26 pp.

Williams, R. (1977) *Marxism and Literature*. Oxford: Oxford University Press.

Williams, R. (1980) 'A defence of realism' in Williams, R., *What I Came to Say*. London: Hutchinson Radius.

Williams, R. (1981) *Culture*. Glasgow: Collins.

Williams, R. (1983) *Towards 2000*. London: Chatto & Windus.

Williams, R. (1989) *The Politics of Modernism: Against the New Conformists*. London: Verso.

Wolfensberger, W. (1985) 'Social role valorization: a proposed new term for the principle of normalization' *Mental Retardation*, 21(6), pp. 254–9.

CHAPTER 10

Power and prejudice: issues of gender, sexuality and disability

TOM SHAKESPEARE

There is quite an industry producing work around the issue of sexuality and disability, but it is an industry controlled by professionals from medical and psychological and sexological backgrounds. The voice and experience of disabled people is absent in almost every case. As in other areas, disabled people are displaced as subjects, and fetishised as objects. A medical tragedy model predominates, whereby disabled people are defined by deficit, and sexuality is either not a problem, because it is not an issue, or is an issue, because it is seen as a problem.

This chapter draws upon three sources. First, existing approaches to disabled people's sexual and emotional lives, which are characterised by the voyeurism and pathological attitude highlighted above. Second, work by predominantly disabled writers, from a social movement perspective, which begins the task of reconceptualising the sexual politics of disability. Third, research being currently conducted by Kath Gillespie-Sells, Dominic Davies and myself, which explores disabled people's own experiences of sex and love through in-depth interviewing.

It would be fair to say that issues of sexuality, relationships and personal identity have been neglected within the disability studies perspective, and it is this absence which we aim to rectify. It is not just that 'the personal is political', but also that a key area of disabled people's experience has been largely ignored. Both academics and campaigners have de-prioritised sex and love. Ann Finger argues that the disability rights movement has not put sexual rights at the forefront of its agenda:

Sexuality is often the source of our deepest oppression; it is also often the source of our deepest pain. It's easier for us to talk about – and formulate strategies for changing – discrimination in employment, education, and housing than to talk about our exclusion from sexuality and reproduction.

(Finger 1992:9)

This chapter represents work in progress, and marks an early attempt to map out some key issues in the sexual politics of disability and to rectify the omissions in accounts of disabled people's experience. It is not the only version, nor the final version: my intention here is not to offer a comprehensive account of disability and sexuality, but to highlight some of the ways in which sexual and emotional experiences can be disabling for people with impairment, and to prioritise strategies and alliances for working in this area.

Imagery, Identity and disability

Asexual, unlovely, undesirable

Jenny Morris quotes Pam Evans' list of assumptions held about disabled people by non-disabled people. These attitudes include a number which are explicitly focused on our sexual difference:

That we are asexual, or at best sexually inadequate.

That we cannot ovulate, menstruate, conceive or give birth, have orgasms, erections, ejaculations or impregnate.

That if we are not married or in a long-term relationship it is because no one wants us and not through our personal choice to remain single or live alone.

That if we do not have a child it must be the cause of abject sorrow to us and likewise never through choice.

That any able-bodied person who marries us must have done so for one of the following suspicious motives and never through love: desire to hide his/her own inadequacies in the disabled partner's obvious ones; an altruistic and saintly desire to sacrifice their lives to our care; neurosis of some sort, or plain old fashioned fortune-hunting.

That if we have a partner who is also disabled, we chose each other for no other reason, and not for any other qualities we might possess. When we choose 'our own kind' in this way the able-bodied world feels relieved, until of course we wish to have children; then we're seen as irresponsible.

(Morris 1991:20ff)

I have argued elsewhere that prejudice and stereotype play a critical role in disabling social relations (Shakespeare 1994a). In the realm of sex and love, the generalised assumption that disability is a medical tragedy becomes dominant and inescapable. In modern western societies, sexual agency is considered the essential element of full adult personhood, replacing the role formerly taken by paid work: because disabled people are infantilised, and denied the status of active subjects, consequently their sexuality is undermined. This also works the other way, in that the assumption of asexuality is a contributing factor towards the disregard of disabled people. There are clear parallels with the situation of children and older people.

Beth, a professional woman with MS, told us:

I am sure that other people see a wheelchair first, me second, and a woman third, if at all. A close friend assumed that, for me, sex was a thing of the past. I think that this is a view shared by the majority. It may have little reality, but influences my self-image.

Our respondents report a failure of professional services to take their sexuality seriously, and an absence of work around sexuality in the disability movement itself. Many social groups face oppressive assumptions about their sexuality – for example, the image of predatory black masculinity, or promiscuous gay male sexuality – but I would argue that stereotypes of disabled people are among the most deep seated and debilitating. Thus, just as public displays of same-sex love are strongly discouraged, so two disabled people being intimate in public will experience social disapproval.

Disabled people themselves often reported serious problems with self-image, having been socialised to think of themselves as asexual or unattractive. Sexual confidence is so centrally about beauty, potency and independence that disabled women and men feel undermined:

I find it hard to switch roles from one who must accept the kind of help that I need, to one who is confident with personal relationships and still able to feel attractive.

(Professional woman)

Other respondents were depressed about being overweight and unfit, as a result of using wheelchairs, and many people had felt ugly at various times of their lives. The narrow concepts of physical beauty within western culture are oppressive to people with impairment: many respondents reported feeling unlike the conventional notion of young, and sexually viable people. Nancy Mairs has written about her physicality:

My shoulders droop and my pelvis thrusts forward as I try to balance myself upright, throwing my frame into a bony S. As a result of contractures, one shoulder is higher than the other and I carry one arm bent in front of me, the fingers curled into a claw. My left arm and leg have wasted into pipe stems, and I try always to keep them covered. When I think about how my body must look to others, especially to men, to whom I have been trained to display myself, I feel ludicrous, even loathsome.

(Mairs 1992:63)

However, she nevertheless maintains a positive self-image: like many of the people we spoke to, she accepts her appearance and is able to feel positive about her looks for much of the time. A man with neuromuscular impairment in our survey reported prejudiced responses from peers at school to his gait – his arched back and thrust-forward chest were mocked, specifically because his appearance suggested he had a womanly bust.

Cultural representations of disabled people in, for example, film and television are a major contributing factor to the negativity surrounding disabled people's sexuality. Cumberbatch and Negrine found that almost twice as many non-disabled characters as disabled characters were depicted in sexual relationships on television drama, and that disabled characters were less likely to have potential relationships. (Cumberbatch & Negrine 1992:66,79)

Gender stereotyping

Gender identity and disabled identity interact in different ways for men and women. Jenny Morris suggests:

The social definition of masculinity is inextricably bound with a celebration of strength, of perfect bodies. At the same time, to be masculine is not to be vulnerable. It is also linked to a celebration of youth and of taking bodily functions for granted.

(Morris 1991:93)

The idea that masculinity involves a denial of weakness, of emotions, and of frailty is very common in cultural criticism. A typical theme in films about disabled people is of the man, often a war veteran, coming to terms with loss of masculinity through impairment – and this is usually characterised or crystallised in the context of impotency or sexual incapacity. Thus *The Men, Born on the Fourth of July*, and *Waterdance* all centre on the disabled man and his difficulties in adjusting. The messages here are about stereotyped male heterosexuality, and stereotyped disabled people's dependency. Prevailing images of masculinity, and of disability, offer conflicting roles and identities. The disabled anthropologist Robert Murphy supports these assumptions:

The sex lives of most paralyzed men, however, remain symbolic of a more general passivity and dependency that touches every aspect of their existence and is the antithesis of the male values of direction, activity, initiative and control.

(Murphy 1987:83)

However, the reality for disabled men is sometimes very different. One respondent, a working-class man with spina bifida, explained to us how his impairment was no barrier to behaving as a typical young man:

I was involved in a lot of fights outside school, although I would never fight a disabled person. A lot of people took the piss out of me, and my brothers had taught me from an early age about fighting. I was in a position where people would take the piss out of me and I would fight back . . . I gave people good hidings! It wasn't a problem that I was in a wheelchair, in fact it was an advantage. I couldn't do anything, and then they would come closer, and then I would smack them in. I would put myself into a position where I knew someone would attack me, and then I would hit them, and feel justified in hitting them . . . I had all these problems at school, they thought my dad was abusing me, I would go in with a black eye and I had been fighting in the streets, and they couldn't accept a disabled person had been fighting.

Sexist stereotypes of women reinforce prejudices about disability: Oliver argues 'there are strong links between the assumed passivity of disabled people and the assumed passivity of women.' (Oliver 1990:72) In both cases, dependency, vulnerability and frailty are the dominant associations in patriarchal culture. Therefore disabled women are represented, as Morris points out, in particularly negative and passive ways (Morris 1991:97) Two American women have written of the dichotomy between the ultra-negative, and the ultra-saintly, view of disabled women:

Disabled women are typically regarded by the culture at two extremes: on the one hand, our lives are thought to be pitiful, full of pain, the result of senseless tragedy; on the other hand, we are seen as inspirational beings, nearly raised to sainthood by those who perceive our suffering with awe.

(Saxton & Howe 1988:105)

The dominant notion of disabled people tends to be male. The young, male, white wheelchair user is the classic disabled person. Most films which centre on disability, centre on disabled men. Morris interprets this in terms of the conflict central to the stereotype of disabled masculinity, as opposed to the reinforcement and conventional feminity of disabled women's images. Of course, the reality of the demographic experience of impairment is that most disabled people are older people, and most disabled people are women. But older disabled women are almost invisible in cultural representation, and are among the most negatively valued members of our society.

Beth summed up her feelings about imagery and identity in words which many disabled people would share:

I do not fit the popular stereotype of either gender or disability. This creates a dilemma for me and for other people.

I think this point is central, and stresses the commonality of disabled women and men: while it is certainly true to highlight the importance of gender to the experience of disablement, it is dangerous to draw simplistic conclusions.

Gender differences

Oliver argues that the experience of disabled women has been neglected in recent publications. He quotes Deegan and Brooks:

Despite the attention given to disability in general and certain impairments in particular, one category within the disabled population has received little recognition or study: women. Like many social change movements, the disability movement has often directed its energies towards primarily male experiences.

(Deegan & Brooks 1985:1)

Oliver echoes another study, in arguing that while disabled women cannot enter traditional male employment roles, they are often denied access to traditional female roles, for example motherhood:

Whereas disabled men are obliged to fight the social stigma of disability, they can aspire to fill socially powerful male roles. Disabled women do not have this option. Disabled women are perceived as inadequate for economically productive roles (traditionally considered appropriate for males) and for the nurturant, reproductive roles considered appropriate for females.

(Fine & Asch 1985:6)

I believe this situation is more complex, in terms of gender, and would dispute the suggestion that men have it easier, on the one hand, and that male experience has received more attention, on the other. Masculinity and femininity are in a process of transitional change within western societies, which makes it difficult to generalise about the strategies of individual disabled men and women. The extent of denial, compensation, social acceptance, and the consequences in terms of role and identity are not clear cut. In terms of the research and investigation of these issues, I would argue that there is a considerable amount of work on disabled women, but hardly any on disabled men (see Campling 1981; Deegan & Brooks 1985; Fine & Asch 1985; Keith 1994; Lonsdale 1990; Morris 1989; Saxton & Howe 1988). Women, working predominantly within feminist contexts have quite rightly explored issues of sexuality, imagery, gender identity and relationships, while men have perhaps concentrated on issues such as employment, discrimination, housing, income, and other material social issues. Michael Oliver's monograph (1990) contains eight references to women in the index, and nine to sexism, but none to men.

Feminist critiques of mainstream, or male stream, theory in other areas suggests that 'people' are falsely constructed from a narrowly male model, hence the need to fill in the gaps and explore women's experiences. In the case of disability studies, I am not sure that a false generic has been the prevailing model, and it does seem the case that specific experience of disabled men has been neglected. Jenny Morris provides evidence that some publications have presented a false generic (Morris 1993:90), but generally I think the male domination of traditional disability research has mainly had the effective of leaving gender out of the picture entirely. It seems almost as if disability studies has reproduced the wider split between public and private with which students of gender studies are familiar. The effect of this is that disabled men's experience is under-represented, which is something that our current research is hoping to rectify. It must also be pointed out that the experience of Black and ethnic minority disabled men and women, and of lesbian and gay disabled people, is similarly under-explored.

The responses of one disabled man, Ed, in our survey highlight the complexity of the disability/gender/sexuality relationship: he felt, with many others, that his masculinity was different as a consequence of his impairment:

One of the interesting things, I feel, is that with the exception of gays, males don't get hassle, whereas you suffer a form of sexual oppression as a disabled man. I very much see myself as a disabled man, not as a heterosexual man.

This respondent felt he could, to some extent, identify with the experience of gay men, or women, or Black people, because he had experienced oppression. It was also clear that women saw his sexuality differently, either as absent, or as unthreatening:

I have known girls go out with me because they wanted to look after me, I'm their little baby in a pram, they push me around everywhere, and they weren't open to the idea that I could get turned on. You also get women who come to see you in the pub and come over and start being very friendly and sit on your knee and wriggle and go 'Oooh!' and you think, hang on, you can't do this . . . I'm sure it works the other way as well, men's attitude towards disabled women for a similar thing, they think it's harmless . . . And anyway, I always find it's like, you're supposed to be flattered because this woman fancies you, because they are not disabled, you should be honoured, and that's why I sometimes get really pissed off by non-disabled people.

While there were costs to his heterosexual identity due to being a disabled man, there were also benefits in terms of improved friendships with women:

I was always a good listener, and I was like a big brother figure for those girls who I fancied. When I fancied a girl, I wouldn't tell her. I was seen as a really good guy, you had a good laugh, I would always listen. Most women saw me as a big brother, rather than a boyfriend, and certainly safe.

Other disabled men echoed this experience, while pointing out that the assumption that disabled men were safe, because they would not or could not be violent or abusive was not born out by the evidence.

Disabled people, sex and love

A range of issues are raised by the practical experience disabled people have of sexual relationships. Here some main themes will be highlighted, although there is currently neither the space, nor the available information, to develop a detailed analysis. Unfortunately, the area of parenting cannot be discussed, although other writers have begun to explore this area (Finger 1991). It is critical not to adopt essentialist analyses, where disabled people's sexual problems are seen as being an inevitable outcome of their impairment, or where attention is solely focused on physical incapacity. Our research indicates that the major problems are the outcomes of prejudice and discrimination, not individual deficit. Impact of impairment on sexual function will not be discussed in this context, both because it is the topic of much work elsewhere, but also because it is not the causal factor involved in disabled people's experience of sex and love. That is, we need to replace the prevailing medical model of disabled sexuality, with a social model which is sensitive to what disabled men and women say about their lives, not based on the preconceptions of non-disabled professionals.

Jenny Morris' book about disabled women included a chapter on sexuality and relationships, but failed to include proper discussion of issues for disabled lesbians (Morris 1989). Other major monographs on disability have also focused on majority heterosexual experience. It is critical to understand that disabled people are also lesbian and gay people, and that Black men and Black women, heterosexual or otherwise, may also have different experiences of relationships. Minorities within the disability movement are increasingly demanding recognition of their experiences, and attention to their needs. Research should be sensitive to difference, in the widest sense, and avoid the generalisations and lacunae. Attention to the way that, for example, gay disabled masculinities are experienced is also useful because it highlights the contingent and dynamic state of gender roles, attitudes and behaviour in general.

One example of the relevance of sexuality or ethnicity is in delivery of care and support services. Because disabled people may need personal assistance, they are more vulnerable to the homophobia or racism of care workers entering their homes. It may be difficult to find support in living a preferred lifestyle. Where disabled people need assistance in preparing for sexual encounters, this may be especially problematic. Again, professionals, advisors and counsellors may be insensitive or actively prejudiced, so that people may have difficulty receiving appropriate services.

The organisation of disabled lesbians and gay men, Regard, has campaigned for the rights of disabled people to be recognised in the gay community, and vice versa. This includes activism around issues of independent living, and recognising the homophobia in, often small and parochial, local disabled and deaf communities. Equally, the lesbian and gay community has been slow to recognise the barriers it presents to the participation of disabled people, especially in attitudes around 'the body beautiful' and the prevailing pressure to be young, fit and sexy.

Denial of sex

As discussed above, stereotypes of disability often focus on asexuality, of lack of sexual potential or potency. Disabled people are subject to infantilisation, especially disabled people who are perceived as being 'dependent'. Just as children are assumed to have no sexuality, so disabled people are similarly denied the capacity for sexual feeling or expression. Where disabled people are seen as sexual, this is in terms of deviant sexuality, for example, inappropriate sexual display or masturbation. Derogatory stereotypes concerning, for example, blindness are typical of this tendency. The assumption of essential abnormality is also reflected in traditional academic work: for example, the American sociologist Lemert, who once wrote that 'Little is known of the sex life of the single blind person' (Lemert 1951:134).

The other side of this is that disabled people are often not welcome in contexts where sex is on the agenda. For example, nightclubs and social venues may aim to cater for young people, fashionable people, and beautiful people. Steps, narrow entrances, flashing lights, smoke and loud noise may all prove barriers to disabled people's participation. Even where disabled people find that they can even access the facilities, they can encounter prejudice which is just as disabling: disabled people are seen as 'not sexy' and are often barred from entry. This experience is common in both gay and straight facilities. At least two of our respondents had experienced exclusion from venues, either on the pretext that their wheelchair constituted a fire hazard, or because their impairment was alienating to other customers. Kirsten Hearn has written of the barriers which the lesbian and gay community presents to disabled people (Hearn 1988:1991).

Policy and provision around disability often neglects to consider sexuality as one of the basic human needs. While housing, transport, education and other needs are dealt with, albeit inadequately, consideration of social and sexual factors is not high on the welfare agenda. Disabled people in day centres or residential homes are often denied privacy, or the opportunity to form emotional or sexual relationships. This failure to prioritise matters which are highly significant to most adults, including most disabled adults, reflects a failure to consider disabled people as fully human. Just like elderly people, disabled people are not seen as having sexual needs, and provision consequently neglects this. Neither disabled people nor elderly people are fully gendered. The typical situation of providing three public lavatories, for gentlemen, ladies and disabled people is a symbolic representation of the degendering to which disabled people are subject.

Another factor involved in the unwillingness to contemplate disabled people's sexual subjectivity is the fear of disabled people joining up with other disabled people, and breeding more disabled people (Humphries & Gordon 1992:100). In a century which has seen repeated policies of eugenics, and ongoing concern about racial purity, the spectre of more impaired children is viewed with alarm. One respondent told us a relevant anecdote:

I heard there was these two people in the supermarket, and they were both wheelchair users, and they had a kiss, I don't know why they wanted to kiss in a supermarket, but they did, and somebody came up to them and said 'Do you mind, it's bad enough that there are two of you.'

This prejudice may be about racial and national purity, or due to cost arguments focusing on the 'increasing burden' to health and social services from this 'deviant' and 'dependent' population. Clearly these fears are subjective and irrational, and can be connected to fears of miscegenation. The Human Genome Project will increase the pressure on carriers of 'defective' genes not to reproduce, or to terminate affected pregnancies. In this context, it is worth pointing out that most impairment in western societies is a product of accident, disease or the ageing process, rather than of defective genes.

Difficulty in finding partners

Disabled people may face barriers in their leisure and social lives, which can be a major obstacle to accessing the environments where non-disabled people make contacts which lead to sexual encounters or romantic relationships. Inaccessible public transport, inaccessible pubs and clubs, and inadequate income can all prevent involvement in the interactions taken for granted by non-disabled people. Where venues do not prevent barriers, people have found themselves excluded because 'cruising' is based on eye contact, and they have visual impairment. Alternatively,

Whilst lesbians with different disabilities who are sighted may be able to do some of this 'eyeing-up stuff', the possibility of them being able to swagger suavely across the dance-floor in their wheelchairs or on their crutches, with their sticks or calipers, is pretty remote.

(Hearn 1988:50)

Lack of access to paid employment leads to exclusion from the workplace, an area where many relationships are initiated. Prejudice, as outlined above, cannot be underestimated. The gay male community, for example, has a major focus on the body beautiful, on dancing and recreational drugs. Respondents also report increasing 'body fascism' in the lesbian community. Such a 'scene' may be inhospitable or unwelcoming to disabled people. Clubs may be in basements or other inaccessible buildings, and many gay men meet in saunas or at public cruising grounds, which may again be inaccessible or unsafe for disabled people. Lesbians increasingly meet for outdoor or sporting activities, which may deter disabled participants.

Possibilities such as phone lines and lonely hearts columns may be an alternative option. However, these may be inaccessible to people with visual or hearing impairments. Moreover, the language of such advertisements is often romanticised, in terms of attractive people, with luxurious lifestyles and high sexual desirability, including physical attributes. This tendency is exaggerate strengths and play down the very human faults and failings of the advertiser may be a deterrent to disabled people, who may feel their impairments will disqualify them from involvement in such negotiations. Alternatively, careful information management is required in the early stages: Bill, a gay man who has met lovers via adverts, pointed out, 'I also can't imagine many replies to letters if you are 100% honest, and say "Oh, by the way I take fits".'

One area where these problems are minimised is in the personal advertisements section of disability-related publications, such as *Disability Now*, which has a large range of disabled people seeking penfriends, friends, lovers and partners. Our current research examines whether disabled people are turning to such sources of social contact because conventional leisure and social environments are inaccessible, because they have experienced rejection in non-disabled settings, or because they are specifically seeking disabled companions.

A danger of such advertisements, and for a range of other contexts designed to enable disabled people to make sexual contact, is that some non-disabled people are seeking disabled partners for reasons which can only be described as exploitative. This may be less malign, in terms of people who are looking for others to care for, perhaps due to personal feelings of inadequacy. A gay man involved in our current research found that respondents to his personal advertisement in the gay press included men who wished to look after him. A more dubious motive is represented by those people, usually men, who are interested in disabled people for fetishistic reasons. There is a considerable voyeuristic interest in disability:

I had some woman who asked me a while ago, what was sex like with a disabled person, I said it's just like sex with a non-disabled person, only ten times better. That was my way of answering them, I thought piss off. Because there's this kind of freak element, it's like, I wonder what it's like doing it with a black person or whatever, it's that kind of thing. You're like a freak show, you're a novelty.

(Heterosexual man)

For example, amputees may be sought after for reasons of sexual taste. I will suggest later that such encounters may sometimes involve abusive relationships. Clearly, these involve power differentials – men exploiting women, adults exploiting children.

A strong parallel could be drawn between these issues, and the popularity of sex tourism, where, for instance, western men go to South East Asia looking for available women and children for sexual gratification, or the practice whereby western men marry women from Asian or Pacific countries, because supposedly 'submissive' and 'vunerable' women are more satisfactory than more 'liberated' westerners.

People who become disabled later in life may find that impairment interferes with the social networks, and personal relationships, in which they are involved. The psychosexual consequences of impairment are among the most difficult of consequences of traumatic injury or disease. Evidence suggests that in heterosexual contexts, disabled men are more likely to maintain their relationships, while disabled women are more likely to find themselves abandoned by their erstwhile partner. One of our respondents suffered extreme unhappiness and jealousy, because her partner took other lovers, because 'he wanted to make love to a woman who could open her legs properly'. She felt trapped, because she depended on him as her main carer:

I cannot describe how awful it feels sometimes, to have to allow a man who insists that he loves, and must see, another woman, to put me to bed, turn me over at night, get me up in the morning, or carry out any of the other tasks that are essential.

Her husband said he could not leave her because 'he thinks he can meet my physical needs better than anyone else'. If she had been non-disabled, she would have left and started again, but did not now feel able to do this, both because of her physical dependency on her partner, but also because she 'did not believe anyone would want me as I am'.

Experience of abuse

While to many people it may seem unthinkable that disabled people should face abuse, it is quite clear that both children and adults face a disproportionate level of physical and sexual abuse. Studies have found a variety of risk factors involved. Typical suggestions are of a double likelihood of having survived abuse. Deaf people and people with learning difficulties are particularly subject to such exploitation. Helen Westcott's research for NSPCC reviews much of the available literature and reinforces these findings (Westcott 1993).

Abuse of children is very likely to come from known people. A significant minority of boys experience abuse, and abuse has been shown to come from both men and women. Child sexual abuse should be seen in the wider context, both of other forms of abuse, but also of abuse persisting into or originating in adulthood. For disabled people, abuse may be normalised. For example, David Thompson has researched cottaging behaviour of men with learning difficulties and discovered abusive relations prevailing in this specific adult context (Thomson 1994)

There is a debate to be had about levels of disclosure, and about availability of research into this area. It is clear that higher levels of abuse are evidenced: I want to look at some of the factors involved. Merry Cross, a disabled activist in this area, has written movingly about this.

'Do you really expect us to believe that anyone could want to have sex with a smelly shitty child like you?' If a (defence) lawyer can speak this way to a disabled child in the witness box at their abuse trial, where can we turn to block out the din.

'This is probably part of some rare syndrome.' If a doctor can write this on the case notes of a disabled girl on whose body he has just noted anal and vaginal tearing and bruising, where can we go to heal our wounds?

(Cross 1994:163)

I do not want to suggest that disability causes abuse. Disabled people are the same as other people. We do not have special needs, we have the same needs. Disabled children do not experience special abuse, they experience the same kind of abuse. But, because of the social context, and the social opportunity, they may experience quantitatively more abuse.

There are the ones who are chosen because they cannot speak of the horror. There are the ones who are chosen because they cannot run away, and there is nowhere to run. There are the ones who are chosen because their very lives depend on not fighting back. There are the ones who are chosen because there is no one for them to tell. There are the ones who are chosen because no one has even taught them the words. There are the ones who are chosen because society chooses to believe that, after all, they don't really have any sexuality, so it can't hurt them.

(Cross 1994:165)

In the rest of this section, I highlight some of the issues which make disabled people more vulnerable to abuse: these I will typify as communication, institutionalisation, dependency, insecurity, invasion, assumption and justification.

First, there is the vulnerability that comes from being unable to communicate what is happening, or what has happened. This means that intervention and prevention may be forestalled, and it also means that abusers will be more likely to choose such a person to abuse.

By communication, I am not just referring to communication impairments, but also to the fact that disabled people may be less likely to be believed. Assumptions, which I will explore later, may cause denial and disbelief on the part of carers and guardians. A blind woman in Westcott's study said:

I don't think it occurred to people that it would happen to a disabled child, and I think that was very marked in that my sister's abuse was investigated but it just didn't occur to anybody to ask me, and I was powerless to say I mean I was in the room sometimes when they'd be talking and I just couldn't say anything for fear of getting slapped or whatever after.

(Westcott 1993:18)

Another woman said: She chose me . . . probably because I had no one else, probably she knew I wouldn't tell anybody. (Westcott 1993:19)

But of course, these issues of communication and belief are exacerbated in certain situations. These are instances where specific barriers to communication exist, and where staff or carers are unable to respond to signals of distress. Disabled people may not share communication systems with adults or nondisabled workers, which may preclude effective disclosure, or disabled people may lack the vocabulary to describe their experiences. Thus all statistics suggest that two groups of disabled people are particularly likely to experience abuse, namely people with learning difficulties and deaf people. Those who have no speech are among the most vulnerable targets of abusers. A further point relates to the possibility of disclosure. A range of non-vocal behaviours is taken as indicative of prior experience of abuse. These may include behaviours – such as inappropriate sexual display or masturbation – which, in the case of people with learning difficulties for example, are explained by carers or staff as normal and typical, and are not problematised as symptomatic of abuse.

Disabled people are more likely to live in segregated situations, and to be institutionalised. Quite clearly, this cannot be taken for granted, but has to be understood in the context of government and local government policy, and the provision which is made for integrating disabled children. Institutionalisation has been analysed by a variety of writers, from Goffman onwards, and we are familiar with the consequences of such contexts. For example, depersonalisation; lack of autonomy and choice; lack of communication with the outside world. Institutions, whether boarding schools, prisons or residential homes, are places where bullying and intimidation takes place more than it does in the outside world. There is more opportunity for victimisation, and given the regimes of power which normally persist, hierachies and pecking orders contribute to the vulnerability of the youngest, the lowest or the most impaired. It is essential to realise that we are not just talking about the abuse of disabled people by staff, carers, ancillary staff and so forth, we are also talking about the abuse of disabled people by disabled people.

A review of the American literature on the institutional abuse of children suggests this is endemic and suggests:

> for example, care workers may use unacceptable forms of restraint, by overmedicalising, or over-feeding children; programmes may abuse children by providing inadequate supervision, monitoring and quality control; systems may abuse by allowing children to 'drift' into care or by failing to monitor the number of changes in placement they experience; society abuses children in care by failing to formulate coherent philosophies, policies and procedures regarding the purposes of care.
>
> (Hardiker 1994:258)

This aspect of disabled people's experience adds to the wider calls for institutionalisation to be abandoned, and for resourced and supported independent living to be made a reality for disabled people in Britain.

Disabled people may be more reliant on others for various physical tasks or social activities. Disabled people may be weaker, and less able to physically defend themselves or run away. Disabled people may be medicated or drugged or even unconscious. Disabled people may need to be bathed, clothed, toiletted, and may need to take taxis or have personal assistance to travel. These factors may contribute to the vulnerability of disabled people. Disabled people may have a variety of carers, because of institutionalisation, fostering, respite care or other processes, and no stable family context. One study found an average staff turnover of 32.8 per cent in public residential facilities and 54.2 per cent in private residential facilities in the United States (quoted in Sobsey & Doe 1991). There may be no access to independent income, or income may be so low as to prevent security. Children with disabilities have been shown to be much more likely to be sexually abused by a surrogate care than non-disabled children (Kelly 1992:164).

It is important to stress the difference between physical dependency and social dependency. Reliance on others is not necessarily about dependence. Access to services delivered as of right, or the financial independence to employ one's own carers can ensure high levels of social independence, despite low levels of physical independence. In current contexts, however, lack of social and physical independence may make disabled people more vulnerable, and may reduce the likelihood of them making complaint of disclosing abuse, especially when abuse is coming from a carer or worker. Many disabled survivors of abuse have kept silence because of the fear of repercussions, which is more critical for those who are institutionalised or dependent.

Disabled people are used to having their privacy and their physical space invaded. This happens as a result of institutionalisation, it happens as a result of infantilisation, it happens as a consequence of physical dependency and inappropriate caring interventions, and it happens as a result of medical examination and treatment. Many people have talked about the way they were paraded naked in front of medical students or other doctors, prodded and pushed and humiliated. A woman with polio linked her frequent hospitalisations as a child to her vulnerability to abuse:

The medical experiences I had made me very vulnerable to being abused it just seemed the same as everything else that had been done to me, so I wasn't able to discriminate . . . there's no way you can say no to what a doctor does to you, they just damn well do it when you're a kid and you don't have any choice about it . . . What the doctors did, they lifted up my nightdress, they poked here and they pushed here without asking me, without doing anything, but in front of a load of other people it was absolutely no different. I didn't say no to any doctor, the porter actually was to me doing absolutely nothing different at all that every doctor or nurse had ever done.

(Westcott 1993:17)

This quotation shows that the process of medical examination is deeply invasive, and disabled people are not considered to be bothered about this. Talcott Parsons (1951) suggested that the sick role enables doctors to ask personal questions and make intimate examinations without embarrassment or other problems. In fact, evidence reveals the medical encounter to be a power relationship with oppressive repercussions. The coldness and formality, the lack of privacy, the objectification of the patient, the lack of communication and the voyeurism constitute a form of violation, not a legitimate procedure. This state of affairs can undermine a disabled person's feeling of ownership and of the body. One woman with a progressive impairment told us:

The more disabled I get, the more my body becomes public property. It is no longer under my control. I must accept intimate help and often lack of privacy if my physical needs are to be met.

Theresia Degener asks, 'If a child has never been allowed to say 'no' to being touched by doctors, nurses or even parents, how can we expect the child, or later the woman, to resist a sexual attack?' (Degener 1992:154)

Given the lack of autonomy and the perpetually threatened integrity of the body, disabled people are often used to switching off, and disassociating themselves from what is happening to the rest of the body. Painful medical interventions or humiliating treatment leaves a legacy of distance and absence from the body. Therapy and surgery may produce negative feelings about one's body. I am not arguing that this makes abuse any easier to deal with. I am arguing that abuse is part of a continuum of oppressive physical and interactional invasion, and that disabled people are socialised into passivity and cooperation. Disabled people are objectified, rather than being seen as people in their own right.

There is an assumption in our society that disabled people, especially those who have high levels of physical dependency or who cannot communicate, are less than human. Social policy has revealed over and over again that institutions and day centres are more like warehouses than welcoming environments. Colin Barnes' book on daycare was called *The Cabbage Syndrome* to highlight this experience. There is another assumption, which feeds into the justifications discussed below, which is that disabled people are not harmed by abuse, that it is less damaging, or that it does not matter. This may influence the likelihood of experiencing abuse, and it may influence the response to abuse on the part of professionals.

Disabled children are patronised and devalued when it is presumed that no one would ever abuse them or it is claimed that, because of their primary and secondary impairments, they do not suffer from the consequences of any abuse which occurs.

(Hardiker 1994:262)

Theresia Degener suggests that 'Disabled women's reports of childhood abuse and rape are much more likely to be assumed to be the products of their fantasies.' (Degener 1992:153) She also draws attention to the fact, discussed above, that disabled people are assumed not to have sexuality, and to be incapable of sustaining a sexual relationship, or alternatively that their sex life is animal-like and brutish.

A range of justifications build on these assumptions. For example, there is the idea that any sexual contact is better than nothing, and that disabled people will not have the opportunity of sexual activity in any other context. Abusers have been able to justify their treatment of disabled people on the grounds that they were doing them a favour, and that no one else would want to have normal sexual contact. There is a wider justification for abuse of disabled people, in terms of the fear and hatred that nondisabled society has for disabled people. There is a tendency to hate those who are perceived as weak; to oppress those who are threatening; to pick on the underdog. I think those without social power or those who are insecure prey on other people who they perceive as inferior to them, and replicate their powerlessness and hurt on these lesser victims.

Sexual abuse of children should be seen in the wider context of multiple forms of abuse against all disabled people. This approach is essential if we are to gather an accurate picture of the experiences of disabled boys and girls, men and women. An example of this is provided by the case of the Outsiders Club. This was supposedly a charitable organisation, helping adult disabled people to meet other people with a view to forming relationships, specifically sexual relationships. The experience of disabled women was that this process, under the banner of sexual libertarianism, was a pretext for men with a fetishistic interest in specific examples of impairment to have access to women in highly abusive contexts. Very rarely was it a case of disabled men meeting non-disabled women, or indeed other potential connections (Rae 1984)

A key aspect highlighted by this example is the issue of power. While specific services and therapeutic interventions may be essential to deal with the individual harm resulting for abuse of disabled children and adults, the key to ending this hidden damage lies in the empowerment of disabled people, the recognition of disabled people as a minority group with equal rights, and the full integration of disabled people into society.

Disability and delight

An account which focuses solely on the very real dangers of abuse and experiences of barriers runs the risk of once more presenting sexuality as a problem for disabled people. Therefore it is important to state that issues of power and discrimination notwithstanding, our research shows that positive and fulfilled sexual lives are a reality for increasing numbers of disabled people.

For example, the development of a positive disability identity, and the opportunity for social exchange presented by the burgeoning disability movement, has opened up many possibilities. Many disabled people are ending their isolation by their political or cultural activism, and are forming strong and happy relationships as a result. Many people spoke of an initial tendency to avoid other disabled people, and to seek non-disabled partners. However, this had been reduced in the case of people who had 'come out' as disabled, and developed a positive identity. The fact that other disabled people would understand their experience of social oppression was a key benefit for people seeking disabled partners.

Even segregated environments could be seen as having some positive benefits, in terms of bringing disabled people together outside the normal constraints of family and home. Thus a number of respondents had attended a residential further educational establishment, where sexual relationships were an unofficial but accepted feature. Ironically, an institution which in other ways was limiting possibilities for integrated mainstream opportunities, was providing, to some, sexual and emotional benefits.

Other respondents talked about the benefits to their sexuality resulting from their impairment and physical lack. For example, one disabled woman talked about her lack of inhibitions consequent on her physical experiences of MS. She felt that her sexual life was more varied and interesting, that she was more likely to initiate sex, and that she had been liberated by having been able to accept her physical difference: her sexual partner also felt freer, and under less pressure to 'perform'. Similarly, people made a comparison with the development of safer sex, which had shifted attention from penetration, to more diverse and varied sexual contact, including touch, massage and other areas of the body. Because people were not able to make love in a straightforward manner, or in a conventional position, they were impelled to experiment and enjoyed a more interesting sexual life as a result.

The suggestion that there may be distinct advantages to disabled sexuality runs against the assumptions of the sexological literature, and the obsession with erection, ejaculation and orgasm which have defined responses to disabled people's sexual 'problems'. It may also suggest that for these heterosexual and homosexual disabled couples, sexual relationships may potentially be more balanced, more equal and more open than for non-disabled people.

Disabled people, and people with HIV and AIDS

Moving forward in the area of disability and sexuality is about prioritising the issue, finding out the reality, and highlighting the problems of exclusion and exploitation which many disabled people face. But it is also about making alliances, and recognising that other groups face similar barriers to disabled people.

Disabled lesbians and gays, who have received negative treatment from the gay and lesbian community, have seen the response to the AIDS epidemic as being hypocritical. On the one hand, lesbians and gays have reacted effectively to the threat, developing education strategies, safer sex, and also raising money for those affected by the virus. On the other hand, clubs and venues have remained inaccessible, and have excluded people who are visibly affected by disfiguring or impairing symptomatic illnesses. Meanwhile, HIV/AIDS is prioritised, while other conditions (including illnesses affecting lesbians, such as breast and cervical cancer) are ignored. Hearn has highlighted this problem:

Those who do recognise AIDS as the biggest threat faced by the gay community for many years may still not recognise the relevance of positive action on the disability front. Like AIDS, disability can strike out of the blue. A car smash, a sudden illness, a knife attack or HIV – all can cause disability.

(Hearn 1991:37)

Her experience is that both the disability community, and the lesbian and gay community have ignored these connections, which is problematic:

Unless the community welcomes all of us, irrespective of our race, gender, class, size or age, it will not be providing a safe and welcoming environment for those sections of the communities whose participation will be threatened because they have AIDS.

(Hearn 1991:38)

Here is an area where disability and sexuality come together in a complex way, and where activists around both issues can cooperate to mutual advantage.

Elsewhere, I have discussed the ways in which HIV/AIDS is a disability issue: for example, because it is medicalised; because people with HIV/AIDS face the same inadequate invalidity benefits as disabled people; because we face the same issues around independent living and control over appropriate care services (Shakespeare 1994b). People with HIV/AIDS face the same patronising assumptions, the same burden of charity provision and representation. Most obviously, the people who live with AIDS/HIV are silenced in discussions about the condition, and lack a voice in decisions about provision and treatment. All these experiences are familiar from a disability movement perspective.

In America, civil rights legislation has benefited people with HIV/AIDS, as well as disabled people: the recent film

Philadelphia culminated in the use of Rehabilitation Act Section 504 to counter the discrimination faced by the protagonist with AIDS. In Britain, organisations of people with AIDS have joined with the disability movement to demand more resources, and full civil rights. This alliance, bringing extra numbers, a new immediacy, and many skilled advocates, will benefit the disability movement immeasurably: John Campbell, chair of the self-organised UK Coalition of People Living with HIV and AIDS, has written: 'Our interests, and the interests of the larger disablement movement are similar in many ways – we have common causes and each movement has much to learn from the other.' (Campbell 1995:5) Of course, many people with HIV/AIDS do not identify as disabled, because they retain a medical model approach to disability, and are not familiar with the new social analysis. Further campaigning and outreach is necessary to share these insights, and build a powerful alliance that can bring about change. Organisations such as ACT-UP, REGARD, and the UK Coalition are at the forefront of these developments.

An interesting theoretical reflection on processes in America and France which parallel these British developments has recently been provided by Paul Rabinow, a leading commentator on the work of Michel Foucault. He refers to work by Daniel Defert, a French AIDS activist (and, incidentally, long-term partner of Foucault, who himself was disabled by AIDS), who suggests:

. . . the pandemic has been the crucible for a new type of social reformer – embodying a new ethical relationship to himself, to others and to things. What we now call PWAs . . . have invented a new patient, one who demands a specific autonomy and a specific set of powers.

(Rabinow 1994:60)

Rabinow further discusses the Human Genome Project, and the way that science and social science are having to take account of each other. Following C. P. Snow, he suggests:

. . . it is neither the technicians nor the humanists alone who will forge a new ethic of truth, suffering and solidarity. The new ethics is emerging from a Third Culture, one Snow did not anticipate, one forged by all those patients at risk, passionately curious about their health, happiness and freedom – us.

(Rabinow 1994:63)

Rabinow fails to notice that disabled people have been forging such an ethic, and such a subjectivity, since earlier than the AIDS epidemic first came to consciousness, and that activism around the new genetics, around HIV/AIDS, and around definitions of normality are central to the disability movement.

Conclusion

Our interviewees were clear about the way forward:

The time for society to work its way round disabled people's sexuality and politics is long past . . . we are not an outer edge of society, we are an integral part of it, and should be allocated all its privileges without any questions or doubts.

(Gay man)

I would like to see those who have power being made to confront their prejudices.

(Heterosexual woman)

Being gay is a natural preference and being epileptic is an unfortunate quirk of fate. It is time the taboo was removed from both.

(Gay man)

Many disabled activists now talk in terms of pride, which is a concept familiar from the lesbian and gay movement:

We have, as disabled people, our own history, we have our own music, we even have our own sport, we have a whole different culture, and that culture is something to be proud of, because our culture has been oppressed for so long, and we are fighting against that in different ways, and I think we should be proud of that.

(Heterosexual man)

The intention of this paper has been to demonstrate issues of power in the context of disabled people's experience of gender and sexuality. I argue that the disabling factors involved in the areas of emotion and sexual expression have been neglected in the analysis of disability, just as progressive positions and the subjectivity of disabled people has been absent from prevailing sexological and medical discourses of disabled people's sexual 'problems'. It is clear to me that research is urgently needed into disabled people's experience of sexual violence and exploitation. I would also argue that research is needed in order to explore the particular experiences of disabled men, of disabled lesbians and gay men, and of gender and sexuality in the context of race and ethnicity. Finally, the incorporation of the experience of people with HIV and AIDS into disability studies perspectives is long overdue, and such an analysis would offer benefits to people with HIV/AIDS, as well as the traditional disabled constituency. Work currently underway seeks to rectify these omissions, and to theorise the relationship between disability and sexuality more effectively and more progressively than has hitherto been achieved. This is an imperative both for disability studies, and for the social movement of disabled people, which is now beginning to take these issues on board.

A Foucauldian perspective on power, focusing as it does on the relationship of power and knowledge, and the immanence of power in discourse, will highlight the nature of unequal power relations in this context. For example, we need to counter those dominant discourses on disability sexuality, which highlight lack and limitation, and develop new accounts based on disabled people's subjective experience. We need to remember that power is a feature of relationships between all subjects, and there are various hierarchies in which people are multiply positioned. Disabled people exploit each other, as well as being exploited by others. When disability comes into play, conventional relationships of gender, age, sexuality and power may become more complex and naunced. We must enable disabled people to speak for themselves, and must recognise that it is the expertise of having lived this experience which is needed, not the professional's technical knowledge.

It was Foucault who showed the ubiquity of power, even or especially in sexuality, but he also allowed for the agency of disabled sexual subjects:

As soon as there is a power relation, there is a possibility of resistance. We can never be ensnared by power: we can always modify its grip . . .

(Foucault 1988:123)

References

Brown, S., Connors, D. & Stern, N. (Eds) (1985) *With the Power of Each Breath – A Disabled Woman's Anthology*. San Francisco: Cleis Press.

Campbell, J. (1995) Disabled People International, in UK Coalition of People Living With HIV and AIDS newsletter, 7th edition.

Campling, J. (Ed.) (1981) *Images of Ourselves – Women with Disabilities Talking*. London: Routledge and Kegan Paul.

Cross, M. (1994) 'Abuse' in L. Keith (Ed.) *Mustn't Grumble*. London: Women's Press.

Cumberbatch, G. & Negrine, R. (1992) *Images of Disability on Television*. London: Routledge.

Deegan, M. & Brooks, M. (Eds.) (1985) *Women and Disability: the Double Handicap*. New Brunswick: Transaction Books.

Degener, T. (1992) 'The right to be different: implications for child protection', *Child Abuse Review*, Vol. 1, pp. 151–5.

Fine, M. & Asch, A. (1985) Disabled Women: sexism without the pedestal, in Deegan, M. & Brooks, M. (Eds.) (1985) *Women and Disability: the Double Handicap*. New Brunswick: Transaction Books.

Finger, Ann (1991) *Past Due: a Story of Disability, Pregnancy and Birth*. London: Women's Press.

Finger, Ann (1992) 'Forbidden fruit' *New Internationalist*, 233, pp. 8–10.

Foucault, M. (1988) 'Power and sex' in L. D. Kritzmann (Ed.) *Politics, Philosophy, Culture*. London: Routledge.

Hardikker, P. (1994) 'Thinking and practising otherwise: disability and child abuse' *Disability & Society*, Vol. 9, No. 2, pp. 257–63.

Hearn, K. (1988) 'A woman's right to cruise', in C. McEwen & S. O'Sullivan (Eds) *Out The Other Side*. London: Virago.

Hearn, K. (1991) Disabled Lesbians and Gays Are Here to Stay! in T. Kaufmann & P. Lincoln (Eds) *High Risk Lives*. Bridport: Prism Press.

Humphries, S. & Gordon, P. (1992) *Out of Sight: the Experience of Disability 1900–1950*. Plymouth: Northcote House.

Keith, L. (1994) *Mustn't Grumble*. London: Women's Press.

Kelly, L. (1992) 'The connections between disability and child abuse: a review of the research evidence' *Child Abuse Review*, Vol. 1, pp. 157–67.

Lemert, E. (1951) *Social Pathology*. New York: McGraw Hill.

Lonsdale, S. (1990) *Women and Disability: the Experience of Physical Disability Among Women*. Basingstoke: Macmillan.

Mairs, N. (1992) 'On being a cripple' in L. McDowell & R. Pringle (Eds.) *Defining Women*. Cambridge: Polity.

Morris, J. (1989) *Able Lives – Women's Experience of Paralysis*. London: Women's Press.

Morris, J. (1991) *Pride Against Prejudice*. London: Women's Press.

Morris, J. (1993) 'Gender and disability' in J. Swain *et al.*, *Disabling Barriers, Enabling Environments*. London: Sage.

Murphy, R. (1987) *The Body Silent*, London, Phoenix House.

Oliver, M, (1990) *The Politics of Disablement*. London: Macmillan.

Parsons, T. (1952) *The Social System*. London: Tavistock.

Rabinow, P. (1994) 'The third culture' *History of the Human Sciences*, 7.2, pp. 53–64.

Rae, A. (1984) 'Refusing to be outsiders' *Spare Rib* 145, pp. 18–20.

Saxton, M. & Howe, F. (Eds) (1988) *With Wings, An Anthology of Literature By and About Women with Disabilities*. London: Virago.

Shakespeare, T. (1994a) 'Cultural representations of disabled people: dustbins for disavowal?' *Disability & Society* 9.3, pp. 283–300.

Shakespeare, T. (1994b) 'Disabled by prejudice' *The Pink Paper*, April 1, p. 13.

Sobsey, D. & Doe, T. (1991) Patterns of Sexual Abuse and Assault, *Sexuality & Disability*, Vol. 9, No. 3, pp. 243–59.

Thompson, David (1994) *Men with Learning Disabilities, Sex with Men in Public Toilets: taking responsibility*, BSA Conference paper.

Westcott, Helen (1993) *Abuse of Children and Adults with Disabilities*. London: NSPCC.

CHAPTER 11

The politics of disability identity

SUSAN PETERS

This paper represents a definite shift in my thinking from
twenty years ago when I first became disabled. Until recently, I
viewed disability through the lenses of social injustice and societal
oppression. I committed myself to a disability rights movement in
the United States that demanded unity and strength, derived from
collective identities and promoted in the common experiences
of oppression. Within the last few years, however, I have felt
that something was missing – my sense of self. I began to feel
the need to re/define myself as an individual and to validate
my personal biography of unique lived experiences in multiple
communities – only one of which was my disability network of
political affiliations. I began a search for self-identity that is more
complex and personalised, and more grounded in sense of physical
and psychological self-image than in the political identity that had
previously consumed my thoughts and activities.

In this paper, then, I embark of a sociological journey through
time and politics of disability that is simultaneously personal and
political. I attempt to reconcile the sense of 'twoness' I have felt
in my earlier quest for a political identity of disability at the cost of
a personal identity. My goal is to develop a pedagogy of disability
that would do two things. First, unite thought and action, reason
and emotion, and self and other through teaching people to act
as border-crossers of the personal/political within themselves as
well as across communities within which they interact. This act of
border crossing strives towards a dynamic marriage of personal
and political identities underpinned by values of self love. Second,
a pedagogy of disability must empower disabled people themselves
to become political advocates through a process of developing a
positive self-identity. In this way of thinking the positive personal
identity is a precondition for political identity. Ultimately, I
strive to define a disability consciousness that would drive a
new discourse on disability identity that is preconditional to
political identity and applicable to disabled people as they live
their everyday lives.

To begin, I analyse and critique the contributions that
sociologists have made to study of disability identity. I also
take society to task, by naming cultural symbols and ritual
performances that have dominated and continue to undergird

much of sociological perspectives on disability identity since long before the birth of sociology as a *bona fide* academic discipline. Second, I look at the possibilities for contributions to disability identity in the developing theories of post-modernism, liberal and radical feminist theories, and critical pedagogy. I will argue that these ideologies hold promise for transforming the field of sociology both at the ideological level and at the level of practice and methodology. Third, I will present a liberation pedagogy of disability identity based on self that draws on the ideas of feminists and post-modernists and critical theorists. Finally, I will explore several themes and the issues they raise that might form the basis of this pedagogy. My ultimate aim is to free young people with disabilities by proposing a pedagogy of disability identity that liberates them from oppression – an oppression which I have learned through painful experiences can be both self-imposed through self-limiting attitudes, and societally imposed through cultural beliefs about disability.

Naming cultural symbols and ritual performances

I begin with symbols and rituals because they permeate our lives, 'form the warp on which the tapestry of culture is woven', and because even sociology is a 'ritual form of secular prayer' (McLaren 1993:38). Rituals and symbols interweave history, biology, private/personal and social/institutional life, producing significant rhythms and metaphors of disability. They act not only on individual psyche, but on sociological interactions and ultimately, world views.

From Victorian times, Western fiction and drama have portrayed tarnished images of people with disabilities which mirror and magnify prevalent societal perceptions. Predominant among these tarnished images are characterisations of disabled people as helpless, useless, pitiable, undesirable. They are dependent, incomplete in body and basic expressions of personhood. Disabled women are submissive, asexual, bitter, and full of self-loathing. In short, disabled men and women are victims of societal misperceptions and of their own inability to reject and transcend the prejudice of others. Even Christy Brown's accomplishments (Brown 1954) were ultimately dependent on a benevolent mother. Most recently, the American fascination with AIDS (which was recognised as a disability protected by law in 1990) reveals our continuing penchant for degradation in the movie *Philadelphia*. The protagonist, who has AIDS, is portrayed as experiencing 'social death' (which preceded his actual physical death) due to prevailing prejudice surrounding the illness and its origins.

These cultural symbols are supported by the medical community with its military metaphors – fighting against disability and disease (e.g., the war on cancer) – which essentially envisages those with disabilities as the enemy; an afflicted and alien other which must be stamped out. Cures take the form of 'defenses' and 'aggressive' intervention. Even the women's rights movement has 'fought' for the right to abort a foetus to avoid the 'double burden of a pathetic disabled child' (Asch & Fine 1988:300).

Aggressive interventions take the form of ritual performance in eradication of disability/disease, and are not limited to the medical community. From its origins, special education has segregated, sheltered, and denied opportunities to children and youth with disabilities on the grounds that disability and/or deviant behaviour do not belong in the 'regular' classroom. The disability rights movement has unwittingly colluded in these ritual performances in the United States and elsewhere through reliance on legal mandates. These legal mandates emphasise disabled peoples' political identity as a minority class of oppressed citizens, at the expense of their personal identity as valuable individuals. For example, Public Law 94–142 (Education of All Handicapped Children Act of 1975) was touted by disability advocates as the solution which would end discrimination and segregation of children with disabilities in American public schools. After twenty years, the result has been an ever-increasing number of students identified as disabled and shunted off to special education classes through the government authorised ritual of the IEPC (Individualized Education Planning Committee). These educational rituals, as well as the underlying concept of 'oppressed minority' that provided the impetus for educational rights laws, serve to further the notion that to be disabled is to be victimised. In other words, one must claim the status of a victim in order to sustain a right to participate in the social system. Finally, in society at large, ritual performances such as telethons to raise money for people with disabilities (e.g., the Jerry Lewis Muscular Dystrophy Telethon) further enhanced this image of disabled people as victims who need special care; special being synonymous with separate. This victim status undermines development of a positive personal identity which is ultimately necessary to overcome the political oppression it fights against.

Although the above examples illustrate American metaphors and rituals in genre, institutions, and communities, the United States is not alone in portraying disability as not quite human, both politically and personally. Cross-culturally and throughout recorded history, people with disabilities have been differentially accorded special status – whether as blind shamans with spiritual powers, as martyrs under Islamic law, or as entertainers and spectacles in early European travelling shows (e.g., the Elephant Man).

Over the last century, scholars within academic disciplines have refined these cultural symbols and ritual performances in theories of the 'Other' – perpetuating and reinforcing the idea that certain classes of people, by definition, are not quite human. While the use of the Other as symbol and metaphor is most often attributed to anthropologists, scholars within the discipline of sociology have also used the Other as symbolic embodiment of disability in society. Since the days of the Chicago School of sociology, American sociologists have concerned themselves with the deviant, beginning with study of 'nuts, sluts and perverts'; e.g. Whyte's *Street Corner Society* (Scull 1988). The definition of deviant expanded to include criminals in Durkheim's work. Then, in the 1960s, sociologists turned their focus towards ascribed status of deviants with Becker (1963) and Goffman's (1963) stress on the process and context of deviance. While Goffman's work served to include the disabled as a deviant group worth studying, our addition to the list of criminals, etc. is hardly cause for celebration. At the same time, Goffman stressed the stigmatised person's reaction to deviance, thus eliminating the possibility of 'deviants' themselves as positive/powerful agents of social control.

While theories of social control expanded the definition of deviance as well as the study of contexts within which deviance occurred, social control theory neglected power and conflict aspects which were assumed to be beyond the capacity of the Other as subordinate minority. Although Bowles and Gintis (1976) made popular the notion of conflict, they focused on class conflict, so that individual human agency was left largely unexplained and unexamined.

A shift from victim or object to subject began to occur in the 1970s and 1980s, however, still situated within socially constructed zones of interaction, leading to the criticism that sociology is 'oversocialised'. Labelling theory, social control theory, medical sociology and the study of deviance still cling to the root paradigms inherent in Parson's descriptions of the sick person (Parsons 1977) and Goffman's concept of 'total institution' in *Asylums* (1961). Social constructivism and symbolic interactionism have given the field of sociology vivid ideas of the place of the Other within society. However, the bodily identity, personhood, and transformative potentials of the individuals within that place have not been the subject of inquiry.

One needs to ask, 'How would the course of sociology and its influence on disability studies have played itself out if Mead's classic work had been entitled, "Body, Self and Society"? rather than "Mind, Self and Society"' (Mead 1934). As a social behaviourist, Mead viewed the self as essentially a social structure. He argued that the idea of self derived solely from the context of social relations. He further argued that 'we can distinguish very definitely between the self and the body' and that 'we can lose parts of the body without any serious invasion of the self' (Mead 1934:136). This neglect of the body as an important mediator in transforming social relations (and of its integral relations with notions of self-identity), has led sociologists down the road of deviance and Other as passive object, rather than self-development and accommodation by active subjects. Writing almost 50 years after Mead, Pierre Bourdieu (1977) developed a concept of 'habitus' that brings together what Mead and others have torn asunder. Bourdieu urges us to abandon all theories that reduce people and their social relations to a mechanical reproduction of social roles assigned to them by the group. 'Habitus' constitutes a 'social system of cognitive and motivating structures' and these structures operate within 'systems of durable transposable dispositions' that 'biological individuals carry with them at all times and in all places' (Bourdieu 1977:82). 'Habitus encompasses ideas of structure, agency, free choice and social determinism, but has not been specifically applied to thinking about disability and deviance' (Epstein 1994). Thus, 'habitus' holds promise for rescuing us from the social determinism of earlier sociologists, but to date, it appears as though our manifest destiny lies in the hands of the Other [sic!].

I have taken the time to name disability symbols and rituals, both within society and within the academic disciplines, not only to emphasise obvious prejudices and limited thinking about disability, but to illustrate the consequences. People with disabilities have largely assimilated these tarnished images in society and the academy. Accepting the idea that we are the Other, we continue to search for ways that will garner our acceptance in 'mainstream' society – mostly through political strategies and legal mandates – while at the same time denying our personal and multiple identities.

Our struggle for personal identity shows nascent beginnings, however, in the creation of new language metaphors for the term disabled – physically challenged, alternative learner – and in our assertiveness in naming the Others as 'temporarily able bodied'. Implicit in these new language metaphors is the recognition that to be labelled is to be (de)valued as a person and is an explicit challenge, both of the disability community and of the academy, to come to terms with self.

A few African-American sociologists provide notable exceptions to the above critique, and give us ways to think about disability identity in comparison with race issues. As a sociologist concerned with race, W. E. B. DuBois capsulated the tension between self and Other that results from devaluation in *Strivings of the Negro People*. He wrote:

It is a peculiar sensation, this sense of always looking at one's self through the eyes of others. One ever feels his 'twoness', two thoughts, two unreconciled strivings; two warring ideals in *one dark body* [my emphasis] whose dogged strength alone keeps it from being torn asunder

(DuBois, 1897:194)

For DuBois, the cause of this tension is the *violence* of ideas, the solution an 'enduring hyphenation'.

Writing almost a century after DuBois, Cornel West (1992) further asserts that one of the best ways to control people is to devalue them, and an effective strategy is convincing African-Americans that their bodies are ugly and their intellect is deficient; and I would add, convincing disabled people that they are asexual, that their disability (perceived or real) is their essence – the negative embodiment of their personhood.

As I reflect on my own life, I find it discouraging to consider the many times I have been put on trial, have had my abilities challenged and my disability essentially considered an obstacle to employability and productivity. When I was asked to join a women's advisory committee on gender issues, I wondered what I had to offer, never having seriously considered myself gendered. It was at this point of gender consciousness that I began to feel my 'twoness', recognising that my sense of self had been torn asunder by my focus on the politics of disability identity. In my search for a way out of this dilemma, disability symbols and rituals within society and within the academic disciplines have combined to limit thinking in regard to disability, to ignore possibilities for transformation, and to stultify a search for new theories that would combine new ways of thinking and new ways of acting (or transforming) disability. For this reason, I have focused my search in disciplines outside of sociology, hoping to draw on new perspectives in education and the feminist movement to build a theory and pedagogy of disability that would liberate and inform our consciousness. I turn to a discussion of these alternative disciplines and their potential contributions in the next section.

Potential contributions of post-modernists, feminists and critical theorists to development of disability identity theory

Having discussed disability symbols and rituals and their consequences, I turn to the possibilities for transformation. It seems to me that transformation must begin with a search for modern theories which show promise for creating a liberation pedagogy of 'living' disability that would reclaim our personhood and reject the idea of the Other. My aim is to correct the oversocialisation of sociology by emphasising personal identity with the goal of teaching ourselves new ways of living our lives. Three basic choices confront us in this task: revolt and revenge, accommodation to the dominant societal group, or self-development. First, revolt and revenge tend to increase societal alienation; in the 1960s and 70s groups of Americans with disabilities often used tactics of strikes and sit-ins to call attention to discrimination. While these tactics were very effective in the short run, and resulted in institutionalised legal mandates, these gains were eroded over time by those who found ways to circumvent the law in retaliation for forced impositions. Second, accommodation to the dominant social group is self-rejecting, ultimately negating our own value and asserting the victim mentality.

The third option, self-development, I believe holds the most promise. Essentially, I argue for a re-vision of disability through listening to the voices and experiences of marginalised Others – namely, in Howard Becker's terms, people for whom the label of disability has been successfully applied (Becker 1963). At its heart, this argument urges a sociology of multiple identities for people with disabilities that challenges our objectification and passive acceptance of ourselves as Others that is found in social theories of disability, most notably social constructivism. The voices and experiences of people with disabilities make visible and therefore possible, our self-development.

To begin, I draw from three emerging ideologies that show promise for informing sociological studies of disability: post-modernism (mainly the work of Aronowitz & Giroux 1991), liberal and radical feminist theories, and critical pedagogy.

Post-Modernism

Post-modernism in the context of education has been very controversial because it rejects the traditional canon for a 'popular' canon. Post-modern educators grant the wisdom contained in the traditional canon, but insist that people and groups need to transform knowledge in accordance with their own sociological, historical, and cultural contexts. For students in classrooms, this transformation means curriculum relevant to these contexts, and instruction that incorporates 'difference, plurality, and the language of the everyday as central to the production and legitimation of learning' (Aronowitz & Giroux 1991:187). From this view, education is viewed as a form of cultural politics that is student-centered and where ' "relevance" is not coded as the rejection of tradition but is a criterion for determining inclusion' (Aronowitz & Giroux 1991:15). The cultural politics inherent in post-modernism makes the relations between truth, power, and knowledge problematic by viewing culture as a terrain of struggle, power, and conflict, not as an artifact of social constructs.

Post-modernism also challenges the cultural borders that have been constructed through this process of cultural politics in institutions such as education. Cultural borders are seen as 'historically constructed and socially organized maps of rules and regulations that limit and enable particular identities, individual capacities, and social forms' (Aronowitz & Giroux 1991:119). When applied to disability issues, these borders include attitudes towards disability which disabled people wish to deconstruct, as well as institutional structures such as special education that separate and exclude people with disabilities from their peers.

Due to the characteristics noted above, post-modernism is particularly valuable to disability scholars for several reasons. First, because it encourages new knowledge of disability that is based on the views of disabled people themselves. Second, post-modernism specifically recognises the need for self-learning that builds on these views. In fact, communication among disabled people through writing and reading about their own experiences is central to the formation of new knowledge as set forth by post-modernists. In this way, voices of disabled students, transform for example, debilitating school rituals such as the Individualised Education Planning Committee deliberations.

To illustrate this point, in my recent research in an urban high school with African-American students labelled as learning disabled, I analyse student voice and student journal writing to deconstruct and transform the concept of learning disabilities (Peters, Klein & Shadwick, forthcoming). This research provides powerful examples of resilient students who consciously redefine the concept of learning disabilities for themselves through critical analysis of their own writing assignment and conversations. My analysis of these students' voices portrays students as street-wise philosophers, and as image-makers, who juggle the consequences of being labelled learning disabled. Essentially, these students must engage knowledge as 'border-crossers' between special and general education classes. Specifically, they have learned to manipulate special education rules and regulations that denigrate their personal identities and limit their individual capacities. Conscious knowledge of this ability to manipulate feels empowering to them. One student who had been labelled learning disabled exemplified this new-found sense of power by observing:

If you found out what they're not good at (professional psychologists) and put a label on them they would feel real low because you are messing around with their weakness, and no one wants you to play with their weakness because if it is your weakness you can say too much about it.

(Peters, Klein & Shadwick, forthcoming)

Crossing the border of special and general education means putting yourself in the Other's place – turning the tables, and in the process, developing new ways of thinking about yourself and others. These students' texts shift the locus of power in school relations at the same time that they change our concepts of disability. The act of reclaiming one's own sense of identity and one's place in the social formation of schooling is a form of personal/cultural politics which I shall argue should be a significant focus of study. Basically, post-modernism makes previous assumptions about disability invalid by providing an insider's counterpoint which forces those in the academy with traditional views to justify their previously unchallenged point of view.

Critical pedagogy

The ability of people with disabilities to use the concepts inherent in post-modernism needs to be cultivated at an individual level. Critical pedagogy attempts this cultivation through encouraging people with disabilities of all ages to think critically, use their personal experience to inform their writing, and to raise awareness of disability and its possibilities for positive self-development. Critical pedagogy is defined as 'working toward a critical understanding of the world and one's personal relation to that world'. The success of critical pedagogy is measured by 'the accumulated amount of political, social and personal awareness each student takes from the class, not by the number of converts' (Deever 1990:71).

Critical pedagogy re-establishes the importance of the learner and recognises her/his ability to produce new knowledge in concert with teachers and scholars. (In fact, critical pedagogy recognises students as teachers and scholars in their own right.) It involves re-examining knowledge as enacted through experience, beginning with a critical examination of the values inherent in such practices as labelling and its consequences. At the individual level, this self-examination entails both self-criticism and a commitment to transforming existing problems inherent in societal practices such as labelling and segregation of students into 'special' education classes.

At the level of the academy (namely, mainstream sociology), I argue in some of my earlier work that our struggle for self-identity must entail a re-examination of theoretical discourse – even social constructivism (Peters 1995). First, because this paradigm has failed to effect change in attitudes and beliefs about disability. Second, it is culture-bound and based on consensus. Finally, the sociological discourse has been invented to a large extent by others. Those of us with disabilities who know what it means to be disabled in the most basic sense of the word through our daily struggles with mobility, physical differences and intellectual challenges, must put forward a disability consciousness which drives creative discourse in the academy.

A disability consciousness must evolve through an analysis of cultural borders such as special and regular education on the one side, and contradictions created by existing paradigms of disability as deviance on the other side. Simply put, if we teach young people with disabilities how to become border-crossers at a personal level, the cultural symbols and metaphors prevalent in today's society will begin to disintegrate. Their subjectiveness becomes evident, rather than the supposed objectivity one perceives if one does not take into account the powerful human action involved in border-crossing.

In concrete terms, this synthesis means no less than a struggle for liberation. An ethnophilosophy of disability needs to emerge from this struggle and manifest itself in the field of disability research, characterised by two features: 1) a break with the ideology of the Other inherent in mainstream sociology, and 2) a renewed questioning of: Who is a person with a disability? How does one describe her/him? what purpose is this description meant to serve? It seems to me that the centrality of experience and value-laden concerns inherent in critical pedagogy would be particularly helpful in addressing these features of disability identity.

A noted feminist, Elizabeth Ellsworth, argues that critical pedagogy fails to empower people because it incorrectly assumes equal power relations (between students and teacher) and its principles rest on the 'Utopian' ideal that 'all ideas are tolerated and subjected to rational critical assessment against fundamental judgments and moral principles' (Ellsworth 1989:314). These moral principles, she argues, repress individual voice. In her view, individual voices are conceptualised in terms of self-definitions that are oppositional to definitions constructed by others. However, she insists that feminist voices are made possible by interactions among women within and across race, class, and other differences that divide them. This duality of purpose – empowering individuals and groups – creates a dilemma between cultivating individual voice through self-definition, and the empowerment found in a unity of voices that is needed to overcome inequities and subordination at a class or group level. While critical pedagogy needs to attend to the issues of imbalances in authority that Ellsworth raises, its inherent focus on a dynamic praxis involving growth, change, and interdependence of thought with action provide the tools and opportunity for empowerment at both individual and group levels.

Historically, the work of Paolo Friere (in particular *Pedagogy of the Oppressed*, 1970) is a precursor of critical pedagogy as espoused today by a significant number of educationists. In his concern for the liberation of peasant farmers from subordination through literacy and self-awareness, Friere developed the concept of 'conscientizacao' or conscientisation. This concept entails dialogue that exists in a constant dialectic between action and reflection directed at transforming structures of oppression. The goal of conscientisation is to develop a self-consciousness as a prerequisite to liberation from an oppression which depersonalises, and therefore dehumanises those who are oppressed. The verb form of conscientisation – conscientise – is a word often used by political activists in the disability movement today. Ranga Mupindu, a leader in the disability movement in Zimbabwe, uses the word in reference to members of parliament who must be prodded to enact laws for people with disabilities. But Ranga insists that enacting the law is not enough – members of parliament must 'know', at a deep level of awareness, why this law is necessary. From listening to the context in which this word is used, then, conscientisation seems to refer to:

the process of making values and experience that are most often repressed or hidden, conscious and visible to oneself and others. It has to do with courageously uncovering the pain, making it articulate, reckoning with it, and entering it into the public/private discourse. It is an uncomfortable, demanding process, requiring both thought and action.

(Lawrence-Lightfoot 1994:70)

Any theory, critical pedagogy included, is only as good or as bad as the way it is interpreted and used in practice. Critical pedagogy, it seems, at least gives individuals the basis for confronting values and experiences, for conscientising ourselves and others. We may use critical pedagogy to raise questions about ourselves and others as well as to examine the moral principles behind these questions. For example, one of the basic questions I have asked myself repeatedly is, 'how can we weave our disabilities (if they are disabilities) into the fabric of our lives, rather than reducing them to isolated traits or innate deficiencies?' The above questions must be answered 'because the pursuit of "other" is inextricably linked with sense of self . . . a limited understanding of self continues to restrict scope and possibility' within the study of sociology (Epstein 1994:10). A dialogue among scholars/students that focuses on this question holds the possibility of raising awareness and liberating us from past conceptions and actions that have dehumanised and pacified disabled people.

A further issue regarding voice and self-awareness is the fact that an 'unwillingness to consider the way in which the body is treated on an everyday basis limits our ability to examine issues of identity, personhood, their social construction, and their potential transformation' (Epstein 1994:24). Feminist theory has contributed a great deal on this issue that may act as a starting point for a discourse on body images as they relate to disability identity and positive self-awareness.

Feminist theory

I find a wealth of possibilities for the study of self and body images in the writings of liberal and radical feminists. Feminists are particularly critical of sociology, asserting that the discipline is antagonistic to recognising feeling and emotion as part of sociology's concerns (Humm 1992). Further, Dorothy Smith argues that if sociology cannot overcome its focus on socially constructed interactions, the sociologist must not stand outside the interactions, but must put themselves inside as knower and discoverer of new relations in a dynamic social system.

For feminists, to know one's self entails a pursuit of self-love. This pursuit is difficult for people with perceived disabilities because they cannot love or value themselves as long as they subscribe to tarnished images in society's mirrors. At a deeper level, Andrea Dworkin insists that 'all struggle for dignity and self-determination is rooted in the struggle for actual control of one's body, especially control over physical access to one's body' (Dworkin 1981:84–5). While Dworkin refers specifically to women, the relevance becomes particularly acute for those with mobility differences whose struggle for control and access to their bodies is constant and often involves overcoming pain.

By contrast, sociologists have treated the body as a 'text' or 'social operator' (recall Goffman's earlier work). But feminists argue that it is at the depths of the organic body that social interactions find their resource (Berthelot 1991). In my own life, I have struggled with a body that has no physical sensation below the waist, that has lost its automatic ability to control biological elimination of wastes, and produces painful stimuli. And yet, I still retain the ability to biologically reproduce new life and to control bodily functions and pain through diet, exercise and meditation. I have learned to control my body in these ways through a process of personal experimentation combined with experiences others have shared with me. This control of my body freed me to interact with others physically, emotionally, socially and intellectually. Although I can't walk, I can swim, ride, talk, have emotions, teach; in short, actively participate – through control of my body and how I perceive my body – in diverse social interactions. These diverse social interactions produce the possibility for multiple identities and participation in multiple communities. In this way, my search for self-identity must encompass more than my membership in a political disability rights movement.

One of the points that feminists stress which is particularly prescient for the formation of this kind of personalised disability identity is the slogan coined by Carol Hanisch in the 1970s: 'the personal is political'. I think that what feminists mean by this term, as exemplified in their approach to gender oppression, is that public policies can be crafted from private experience. However, I would argue that private experience must be shared (as in the example of my own experimentation with my body) in order to create a coherent and radical politics of disability. This interdependency between public and private experience has the characteristic of a dialectic: the personal is political, but the political must also be personal. Sheila Rowbotham elaborates on this point, and I quote her assertions at length here because I think they speak directly to the point of the politics of disability identity as it relates to the preconditional need for self-expression:

In order to create an alternative an oppressed group must at once shatter the self-reflecting world which encircles it and, at the same time, project its own image onto history. In order to discover its own identity as distinct from that of the oppressor it has to become visible to itself. All revolutionary movements create their own ways of seeing. But this is a result of great labour. People who are without names, who do not know themselves, who have no culture, experience a kind of paralysis of consciousness. The first step is to connect and learn to trust one another.
(1973:94)

Shattering the tarnished images of disabled people requires this same sort of visibility through self-awareness that Rowbotham is speaking of. Discovering ones own identity is the practice of self-awareness in action, and this discovery is what Paolo Friere and Ranga Mupindu mean by conscientisation, which is the work of critical pedagogy. Connecting and learning to trust each other as people first is the centerpiece of post-modernist popular canon. From these theories we may propose a process for development of disability identity which we turn to next.

The politics of disability identity in action

Taken together, the three emerging ideologies described above create a problem and goal for sociologists who study disability: how to unite thought/action, reason/emotion, self/Other. Further, to combat the paralysis of consciousness that I believe currently exists in the study of disability, I suggest five essential components for a new discourse on disability.

1. The existence of a group of philosophers with disabilities living and working in an intellectually stimulating cultural milieu resolutely open to new possibilities in the lives of disabled people.
2. A substantive and critical use of external philosophical 'reflectors' such as the notion of border crossing, which would promote disability in a universal and cross-cultural framework of thought, necessitating a rethinking of the Other.
3. A selective and flexible inventory of values as they relate to disability – including attitudes, symbols and rituals – which would possibly provoke thought in the sense of building a new socio-political philosophy of disability based on a critical examination of both the past and the future of people with disabilities.
4. A clear dissociation of the sociologist's academic baggage from cultural baggage which would amplify major contrasts (e.g., self versus Other, body versus mind, deviance versus oppression).
5. An examination of sociologists' main temptations – focus on social interactionism without self-examination of a person's place or 'habitus' within the social system.

The tasks described above might begin with a focus on four interlocking themes. The first two – spiritual (religious) and body (organic) images – address personal identity as a self-centred activity. The second two – cultural pluralism and political activism – define and expand personal identity to address the politics of identity formation. Both levels of identity are necessary for a liberation pedagogy of disability to develop.

The Personal Search for Identity

Personal identity as a self-centered activity take place in three major locales: The church, school and family environment. The Judeo-Christian influence is the major religious force in America. However, all cultures practice some form of religion, defined by Geertz as: 'a system of symbols which acts to establish powerful, pervasive, and long-lasting moods and motivations' (Geertz 1973:87). Geertz further asserts that religions clothe conceptions of existence with an aura of factuality that makes these moods and motivations seem uniquely realistic.

Religion is often appealing to many disabled people because it offers other-worldly substitutes for ordinary bodily gratification they desire. (More to the point, religion has been described as a crutch or coping device.) However, religious rituals can be very harmful to the body image and personhood of people with disabilities. Soon after my accident in 1974, I was taken to a group of spritual healers when my physical body was not responding to medical treatment in terms of restoring my spinal cord. I went to placate my mother's friend and spent an hour subjected to praying and laying on of hands. In the end, I was told that the healing had failed because I had a 'bad heart', which I translated to mean a 'bad attitude'.

My friend Rangariru had a similar experience with traditional African healers after he contracted polio in Zimbabwe. As a young child, Ranga was taken to a mountain top where traditional rituals were performed and then left by himself overnight to be 'cleansed'. Throughout his youth, Ranga's mother insisted he attend church. But the priests would use him as a model, start quoting the Bible and saying, 'If you're sick, *you will walk.*' As a result, Ranga ended up saying to himself, 'There's no point in going there. I don't want to go and be embarrassed.'

One further example illustrates the harm that can be done in the name of religion. As a health educator (1974–6), it was my job to visit former spinal cord injury patients at home for follow-up evaluations. One young man had spent two years in bed, waiting to be healed and fully expecting until the day he died that God would perform this miracle cure.

Religion can play a vital role in developing spiritual identities that would provide a reservoir of strength and resources for disabled people's quality of life. However, as the above examples show, it too often serves as a burden/obstacle, conveying long-lasting conceptions of guilt, loss of power and control; and perpetuating the view of disabled people as victims as well as consigning them to a sick role until 'healed'. Schooling enforces similar rituals and symbolic roles in its practice of labelling and consigning people with disabilities to special classes, where they must earn their way back to being normal again. These special classes essentially lead people with disabilities into bondage while promising salvation – but for the vast majority, salvation never comes.

At the level of family, formation of identity and particularly sex-role socialisation have powerful influences on young men and women with disabilities. Parents often discourage or prevent sexual activity, dating and marriage on the part of their disabled sons and daughters. Sterilisation of mentally disabled women (without their consent) is still legal in many countries. These practices are often justified by parents in the guise of protecting/sheltering their 'vulnerable' youth from the 'outside' world, and is said to be 'in their best interests'.

Families may also have a very powerful positive influence on children with disabilities. In my own life, my disability drew my family closer together. We became more expressive with each other in terms of feelings, and better able to express our needs and wants. We spent more time together. We had a heightened sense of the fragility of life, and therefore a better appreciation of the need to spend quality time with each other. I learned patience, and gained a deeper understanding of the sacrifices my parents had made for me not only during the time of my initial disability, but throughout their lives. Because my family supported me, and let me know they loved me in words as well as in the actions of attention, caring and listening, I was able to develop a renewed sense of myself as a valued and valuable person, and I was able to go on and accomplish many significant milestones – including attaining a PhD from Stanford University.

In considering these interrelated themes of body image, religious ontology, and family relations, sociologists and others in the field of disability studies should consider not only the role and function of ritual and symbol, but the 'epistemological vector in the body considered as product and producer, the place of pain and pleasure, alienation and reappropriation, inscription and affect'. (Berthelot 1991:401). Specifically, a pedagogy of disability might integrate these vectors through focus on social persona, developing a consciousness of positive body images, exploring ways in which negative stereotypes of sexuality are internalised, and considering the notion of a continuum of sexual/emotional impulses and the influence of observed and learned behaviour on sexual/personal development (Smith-Rosenburg 1983). This focus is an absolute precondition to socio-political transformation of people with disabilities, for without a solid grounding in who one is as an individual, political identity becomes a window dressing for the tarnished images of others, rather than an internalised set of values based on self-love.

The political search for identity

The second two themes – cultural pluralism and political activism – depend on a positive sense of self and expand self-identity issues to include consideration of the personal as political. I expect my colleagues will have more to say on these issues, however, I do want to make one point. That is, that the disability movement has often insisted on solidarity to advance our human rights. Our own disability community, including scholars of disability studies, needs to forge new relations between identity and difference. As a specific example, diversity is an overused concept which has become trivialised, and in combination with the pressure for solidarity, has thwarted our self-development. In addition, the concept of 'oppressed minority' points the finger at Others, while neglecting our own conceptual weaknesses. Finally, the whole notion of difference is problematic because difference is always perceived in relation to some implicit norm. It perpetuates the illusion that individuals are measured from some universal standard of objective authority.

Despite predominant symbols and rituals which carry negative conceptions of disability, some people with ascribed disabilities choose to embrace their difference as a positive identity marker. They derive power from their differences and assume the role of border-crossers. This identity is often developed in spite of formidable barriers such as the absence of familial role models, the presence of culture-bound ascribed deficiencies, and the religious insistence on miracle cures. For these powerful individuals, the social structure influences without strictly determining beliefs and behaviours. How does this transformation occur? Under what circumstances? The politics of identity and community that I described earlier need closer scrutiny in this regard.

Conclusion

Through a long and difficult process of search for personal identity, I have come to the conclusion that individual perception is intertwined with collective identity, but must remain simultaneously independent of it as well in order to change it. Throughout this paper I have argued for a new disability identity – one that needs to integrate the personal and political in an 'enduring hyphenation'. One identity depends upon the other. I argue as well that these identities must rest on foundations of self-love and spiritual models, as opposed to sociological models that rest on foundations of the 'victim' mentality, deviance, and the Other as passive object. Disabled people have come together in political action groups for their survival/human rights, and in order to develop an ethos unique to the experience of disability. As this ethos develops, it allows room for the individual to self-explore. At first, this self-exploration seems separating and alienating from the group and its societal preservation functions. However, as the individual builds self-awareness, this sets the preliminary stage for a return to group cooperation and therefore carries the potential for recharging group values. Essentially, as group survival is satisfied (through such actions as the Americans with Disabilities Act, for example), group resources become available for individual identity to develop. Each time individuals leave the group (and their political identity), they return and reunite with the group at a higher level of integration, so that there is a constant inbreath and outbreath of stability and novelty essential for individual and group renewal and revitalisation. Individuals, in their relation to the group, must be reasonably independent, however, so that when they come together as a group they are not mutually dependent. When this mutual dependency takes ascendancy, the victim mentality subordinates disabled people to themselves and others.

This movement in and out of personal and political identities also shifts borders. Cultural borders change boundaries, expand, become larger, and then new borders are drawn that produce new problems and require new strategies to meet new challenges.

These notions of multiple identities, their interdependence, and the dynamics of border-crossing involved in creating identities might serve as the focus for sociological studies on disability. This focus will require shedding notions of the Other and the theories of social interaction that negate self/body identities. The five essential components for a new discourse on disability provide the tools for sociological studies about disability. The feminist and educational theories of post-modernism and critical pedagogy provide the framework for these studies. The voices of disabled people themselves provide the voice and the substance/content of the studies as well as the direction they should take. The ultimate goal is liberation through conscientisation.

In the final analysis, though, the act of conscientisation necessitates pushing ourselves beyond discourse and scrutiny to action. The philosopher group I propose must include students such as the African-American street-wise philosophers in my earlier study. We must not only support other scholars, but the future generation of scholars. The message conveyed by these discourses necessitates a dynamic interaction between theory and what goes on in school and at home with a focus on values and self-love. In this respect, the medium is the message and the tools for action. Specifically, building the processes for creative change, goals and strategies for action must be the end result. However, criticism and vision are not static but are in a continuing process of transformation. As we realise our visions, our problems are transformed. This transformation is the essence of a liberation pedagogy of disability necessary for teaching ourselves new ways of living through personal and political processes of identity formation.

References

Aronowitz, S., & Giroux, H. A. (1991) *Post-modern Education: Politics, Culture, and Social Criticism.* Minneapolis: University of Minnesota Press.

Asch, A. & Fine, M. (Eds) (1988) *Women with Disabilities: Essays in Psychology, Culture and Politics.* Philadelphia: Temple University Press.

Becker, H. S. (1963) *Outsiders: Studies in the Sociology of Deviance.* New York: Free Press.

Berthelot, J. M. (1991) 'Sociological discourse and the body' in M. Featherstone, M. Hepworth & B. S. Turner (Eds) *The Body: Social Process and Cultural Theory*. London: Sage Publications, pp. 390–404.

Bourdieu, P. (1977) *Outline of a Theory of Practice*. Cambridge: Cambridge University Press.

Bowles, S. & Gintis, H. (1976) *Schooling in Capitalist America*. New York: Basic Books.

Brown, C. (1954) *My Left Foot*. London: Octopus Publishing Group.

Deever, B. (1990) 'Critical pe ιgogy: the concretization of possibility' *Contemporary Education* 61(pp. 71–7.

DuBois, W. E. B. (1897) 'S ι ηgs of the Negro People' *Atlantic Monthly*, 80, pp. 194–8.

Dworkin, A. (1981) *Pornography: Men Possessing Women*. London: The Women's Press.

Ellsworth, E. (1989) 'Why doesn't this feel empowering? Working through the repressive myths of critical pedagogy' *Harvard Educational Review*, 59(3), pp. 297–324.

Epstein, I. (1994) 'The search for other through the escape from self' Paper presented at the 1994 Annual Meeting of the Comparative and International Education Society.

Friere, P. (1983) *Pedagogy of the Oppressed*. New York: The Continuum Publishing Corporation.

Geertz, C. (1973) *The Interpretation of Cultures*. New York: Basic Books.

Goffman, E. (1961) *Asylums*. New York: Doubleday.

Goffman, E. (1963) *Stigma*. Harmondsworth: Penguin.

Humm, M. (1992) *Modern Feminisms: Political Literary Culture*. New York: Columbia University Press.

Lawrence-Lightfoot, S. (1994) *I've Known Rivers: Lives of Loss and Liberation*. New York: Addison-Wesley Publishing Company.

McLaren, P. (1993) *Schooling as a Ritual Performance: Towards a Political Economy of Educational Symbols and Gestures*. London and New York: Routledge & Kegan Paul.

Mead, G. H. (1970[1934]) *Mind, Self and Society*. Chicago: University of Chicago Press.

Parsons, T. (1977) *Social Systems and the Evolution of Action Theory*. New York: Free Press.

Peters, S., Klein, A. & Shadwick, C. (forthcoming) 'Special education and the "alter-eagle" problem', in B. Franklin (Ed.) *When Children Don't Learn: Student Failure and the Lives of Teachers*. Columbia: Teachers College Press.

Peters, S. (1995) 'Disability baggage: changing the educational research terrain' in Clough, P. & Barton, L. (Eds) *Making Difficulties: Research and the Construction of Special Education Needs*. London: Paul Chapman.

Rowbotham, S. (1973) *Woman's Consciousness, Man's World*. Harmondsworth: Penguin.

Scull, A. T. (1988) 'Deviance and social control', in N. J. Smelser (Ed.) *Handbook of Sociology*. London: Sage Publications.

Smith-Rosenberg, C. (1983) 'The female world of love and ritual: relations between women in nineteenth century America' in E. Abel & E. K. Abel (Eds) *The Signs Reader: Women, Gender and Scholarship*. Chicago: University of Chicago Press.

West, Cornel (1993) *Race Matters*. Boston: Beacon Press.

Whyte, W. F. (1943) *Street Corner Society*. Chicago: University of Chicago Press.

Zola, I. K. (1982) *Ordinary Lives*. Cambridge: Applewood Books.

PART FOUR

Disability: A Particular Research Method

Reading through the chapters in this book you will have been confronted with references to the disabling impact of particular types of research. One of the significant aspects of discrimination is the extent to which the voices of disabled people have been excluded from both academic and popular discourses within society. This is not because they have nothing to say, but rather, it is either a question of being subservient to the significance of professional articulations or not something which a disabled person can be expected to do. These sorts of assumptions reinforce a deficit view, one which ultimately regards those involved as less than human.

The chapter by Booth provides a particular approach to research, one which seeks to give dignity to the disabled people involved. In this account Booth explores the use of narrative methods with people who have learning difficulties. It is concerned with the central question of how to give a voice to people who lack words. He argues that sociologists should experiment with ways of constructing narratives that allow for the role of the imagination and for the use of creative writing as a tool in its own right.

It is important to remember that this is but one, important, approach which sociologists use as a vehicle for research. However, as you will find from your reading of the chapter, it raises several fundamental and challenging issues which need to be seriously and urgently addressed.

CHAPTER 12

Sounds of still voices: issues in the use of narrative methods with people who have learning difficulties

TIM BOOTH

This chapter explores the use of narrative methods with people who have learning difficulties. By narrative methods I mean methods aimed at depicting people's subjective experience in ways that are faithful to the meaning they give to their own lives. I shall argue that sociologists should take their lead from historians by experimenting with ways of constructing narratives that allow more scope for the play of the imagination and for the use of creative writing as a research tool in its own right.

As Bowker (1993) has recently observed, the age of biography is upon us, and narrative methods are poised to regain a central place in sociological research. Two linked arguments have contributed to this resurgence of interest in storytelling – an interest unmatched since the heyday of the Chicago School – and both owe much to the influence of feminist scholarship and critical race theory.

The 'excluded voice thesis' postulates that narrative methods provide access to the perspectives and experience of oppressed groups who lack the power to make their voices heard through traditional modes of academic discourse. The second argument criticises conventional scholarship for subordinating the reality of people's lives to the quest for generalisation. Generalisation involves the loss of precisely the kind of detail that distinguishes personal experience. By contrast, storytelling provides a point of entry into the world of experience through the imagination of the reader. Thinking concretely in narrative terms combats what Connerton (1989) has called the 'forced forgetting' imposed by abstract reasoning. Stories also restore the emotional content of human experience suppressed by objective methods of reporting.

For precisely these reasons, the upsurge in storytelling might have been expected to impact on research in the learning difficulties field. Certainly there has been a growing recognition in recent years of the importance of listening to the people who have been labelled. Ten years ago, Richards (1984) could identify only five British studies in the previous 20 years which had involved people with learning difficulties as informants. This picture has now changed significantly. Numerous studies have been done in hospitals (Booth *et al.* 1990; Potts & Fido 1990; Cattermole *et al.* 1987), in hostels (Sugg 1987; Malin 1983; Brandon & Ridley 1983), in Social Education Centres (Booth & Fielden 1992), in staffed houses and independent living schemes (Flynn 1989; Lowe *et al.* 1986; Passfield 1983) using people with learning difficulties as informants (see also Welsh Office 1991).

With a few notable exceptions, however, very little work has been done using narrative methods and the life story approach. Whittemore *et al.* (1986) found only four truly autobiographical works in their search of the literature. At the same time, they report, biographical material has generally presented only a 'pointillistic interpretation' of its subjects by focusing on isolated character traits or aspects of their lives that happened to catch the researcher's attention. Often, too, the biographical form has been used as a device for recounting the author's (frequently a parent or sibling's) own story. For the most part, the views of people with learning difficulties have been subordinated to other people's purposes. As informants in research they have been used as sources of data for sociologist's narratives rather than regarded as people with their own stories to tell. Consequently, the literature is still largely void of the experience it seeks to portray.

The reasons for this state of affairs have their origins in prejudice. Common stereotypes have helped to shape thinking and attitudes within the research community as surely as in the wider society. People with learning difficulties have mostly been treated as objects of study rather than credited with any integrity as people. They have generally been seen as problems for other people rather than as individuals with lives of their own. The primary focus has been on their deficiencies rather than their capacities (Mount & Zwernik 1988). Such attitudes and assumptions have encouraged the view that the basic tenets of qualitative research do not hold up well in the study of people with learning difficulties. Plummer (1983), for example, suggests that good informants 'should be fairly articulate, able to verbalise and have "a good story to tell"'. Researchers have been too quick to assume that narrative methods are inappropriate with inarticulate subjects. Likewise Spradley (1979) argues that a good informant should be thoroughly 'enculturalised' whereas lore and language have long depicted people with learning difficulties as less than fully human ('subnormal', 'idiot', 'moron', 'imbecile', 'feebleminded', 'retardate'). Life-story research also entails the development of a close and intimate relationship between the researcher and the subject. Perhaps researchers have (more or less unwittingly) been predisposed to find excuses for not engaging too closely with people who have learning difficulties. The fact remains that there is much to commend the use of narrative methods with this group of informants.

The power of narrative

Narrative methods vary in their forms and purposes. The purest form of narrative is the *autobiography* where the subject is also the sole author. *Reminiscence* is the unstructured recalling of past events and feelings without any attempt to be inclusive or thorough about the life course. *Life review* is a process of reflection in which people appraise their own past from their standpoint in the present. The *life story* is a collaborative account of all or part of an individual's life delivered orally by that person to an amanuensis. The *life history* subsumes the life story but also includes biographical information from a range of other sources.

These narrative forms may serve a variety of uses. For example, adapting Abrams (1991) slightly, five overlapping categories of narrative may be identified. *First-person agony narratives* recount painful experiences as a means of challenging the moral or social order through the sympathies or conscience of the reader (see, for example, Ashe (1989) who weaves her own experience of childbirth into an examination of the legal regulation of reproduction). *Insider narratives* aim to provide an insight into subjective worlds beyond the reader's ken (see, for example, Lewis' (1961) classic account of family life in a Mexican slum). *Grounded narratives* render abstract ideas accessible in terms of everyday human experience (see, for example, Williams (1991) on racism). *Fringe narratives* give voice to previously unheard or suppressed perspectives (see, for example, Jane Fry's account of her life as a transsexual in Bogdan (1974) or Parker (1991) on 'lifers'). Finally, *mould-breaking narratives* help to reformulate a problem, cast something in a new light or otherwise change our understanding (see, for example, Warshaw (1989) on the date rape phenomenon).

Despite this variety, narrative methods display a number of common characteristics and strengths.

- They provide an 'inner view of the person' (Birren and Deutchman, 1991) by treating people as 'expert witnesses' in the matter of their own lives whose stories can provide a point of entry into their world through the imagination of the reader.
- They are a means of making abstract claims more tangible by grounding them in concrete lived experience.

- They help to counteract the problem of the 'disappearing individual' in sociological theorising where the search for abstraction and generalisation often renders people into little more than ciphers and leads both scholars and students to lose sight of human individuals as a creative force in the making of their own lives and their own history.
- They form a bridge between the individual and society by giving access through people's lives to structural features of their social world. By 'listening beyond' (Bertaux-Wiame, 1981) the words of any particular informant, it is possible to pick up the echoes of other people's experience and to identify the themes that make them also the stories of a group. These common threads connecting people's accounts reveal how their lives are shaped by the wider society and throw light on the network of social relations to which they belong. In this way, as Ferrarotti (1981) has observed, the 'effort to understand a biography in all its uniqueness . . . becomes the effort to interpret a social system'.
- They help to combat an 'over-determined' view of reality, brought about by methods and modes of reasoning that impose order and rationality on the world, by unmasking the 'confusions, ambiguities and contradictions' (Faraday & Plummer, 1979) that characterise people's lives and everyday experience.

The problem of narrative

The criticisms of narrative methods – including problems of implicit conceptualisation, unrepresentativeness, lack of objectivity, verification, unmanageability, partiality, unreliability – have been well rehearsed in the literature (see especially Allport 1947). It is not part of my purpose to go over the same ground. Instead I shall focus on a specific problem identified by Baron (1991): namely, that those who most need to have their stories heard may be least able to tell them. A particular version of this problem arises directly in narrative research with people who have learning difficulties. How do you give a voice to people who lack words?

I shall illustrate this problem by reference to a recently completed study of parents with learning difficulties (Booth & Booth 1994). The guiding purpose of this study was to provide a parent's view of parenting using the life story approach. A total of 33 parents (20 mothers and 13 fathers) took part of whom 25 (18 mothers and 7 fathers) had learning difficulties. By looking for the common threads in their lives, the aim was to produce an account that is true to the experience of such parents at the level of subjective reality if not statistical description. A full account of the conduct of the study is provided in Booth & Booth (1994).

The life story approach produces data in the form of narrative rather than numbers. As Denzin (1989) says, 'lives are available to us only in words'. The process by which accounts of lives are produced and turned into text is therefore an important methodological issue in this kind of research with implications for the ownership and authenticity of the story as told. This process assumes even greater significance when the subjects in question are unable to communicate fluently in words. Let us explore four aspects of this problem using examples and material drawn from the study of parents with learning difficulties.

Narration

Bertaux (1981) says that 'a good life story is one in which the interviewee *takes over the control of the interview situation* and talks freely' (italics in original). This rarely happened in our study and, except on a few occasions at the first interview, it was usually the partner without learning difficulties who took the lead in this way. Generally speaking, our informants were more inclined to answer questions with a single word, a short phrase or the odd sentence. The following extract from a transcript is not untypical. It comes from the first recorded interview with the parents at which the interviewer was trawling for information about their background and family history:

Int: How long have you been living together, or going together?

Fthr: Well, I come to Wakefield in 1984. I were living in Denby then, weren't I?

Int: And where did you meet each other then?

Fthr: At Centre.

Mthr: Centre. I used to go when Craig (their first child) was born.

Fthr: We had an Autumn Fayre.

Int: Which Centre's this?

Mthr: Sandalwood.

Fthr: Down here.

Int: And you both were there, were you?

Fthr: I used to work there. And we had sort of an Easter Fayre and that.

Mthr: If he goes back there, I can go to their Christmas parties and Easter dos. Because I used to go there before.

Int: And what were you doing? Gardening, you say?

Fthr: Gardening, yes.

Mthr: Because our Trish works there, and her boyfriend lives there.

Int: Is that your sister?

Mthr: Yes, my sister. She works there and her boyfriend works there.

Int: And where were you then when John (*the father*) was working there? Were you living at home?

Mthr: No. I had this house then, didn't I.

Fthr: She was living at home.

Mthr: I was at home.

Int: What, with your mum?

Mthr: No. I had this house when my mam was living, and then she died so I had this house when she died.

Int: And you stayed living in the house? And it was this house, was it? So you were brought up here, were you?

Mthr: No. I were brought up, I were born in Leeds in ambulance, not in hospital.

The extract displays a number of the common characteristics found among the parents in their role as informants. They tended not to speak in long, uninterrupted stretches of narrative. Questions frequently elicited one-word or a simple phrase in reply. Information had often to be gleaned by direct rather than open-ended questioning. They were better able to handle questions about people and places than cope with abstract ideas or make comparisons. They talked more easily about things happening in the here-and-now than about former times or past experiences. Also, their feelings and concerns were more often revealed in their behaviour and their reaction to events and situations than through reflection and analysis.

Although our informants varied in their language skills, their conversation tended to show: an instrumental rather than an expressive vocabulary; a present orientation; a concrete rather than an abstract frame of reference; a literal rather than a figurative mode of expression; a focus on people and things rather than feelings and emotions; and a responsive rather than a proactive style. None of these characteristics, of course, are unique to people with learning difficulties, although the challenge presented to the researcher is perhaps more overt in their case. Most importantly, this lack of verbal fluency was not a barrier to the parents telling their stories. It does, however, have implications for the role of the interviewer (who must expect to have to work harder), the conduct of the interviews (techniques other than just talking have to be used to engage the informant), the length of time it takes to compile a life story (the full story emerges only slowly a bit at a time), and the way it is written up.

The lack of continuous narrative in people's accounts of their experience of parenting made it necessary for the researcher as editor to play a fuller part in the transformation of their stories into text.

Editing

Turning transcripts into publishable text involves a loss of material. In our study this often presented a real dilemma. Parents' conversation generally centred on the everyday, the particular and the here-and-now; and their talk tended to dwell more on things that had happened to them than on things they had done. These features were not adventitious. They expressed the outlook and concerns of people whose vulnerability in the world obliged them to take each day at a time. The form of their stories reflected the form of their lives (Bertaux-Wiame 1981). When Rosie Spencer went on about the doings of her community nurse in interview after interview she unwittingly revealed her subjugation and resistance to the power that professionals wielded over her. Excising repetitions and other material that does not seem to carry the narrative forward inevitably runs the risk of breaking the link between the lived life and the story as told. The editorial task draws narrative researchers ineluctably into betraying their subjects by representing them (while raising the question of how much more is lost by research that fails to engage with the person at all).

Cutting and pasting is the principal method for generating text. Material from different parts of the same interview or from different interviews is spliced together to form a coherent narrative or to develop a theme. For example, the following passage pulls together a series of statements made at different times by the same informant to express her view of social workers (superscripts identify the interview/line number):

'I don't like social workers on my back. I hate it$^{1/136}$. (I)'m sick of hearing them, do this, do that. I'm not one years old. I'm 26 now$^{1/3\&4}$. (T)hey interfere with us$^{1/140}$. I can manage my own$^{1/4}$. I just don't want any help, that's all$^{1/174}$. I want to get rid of them. I don't like them being on my back and my mam don't like them$^{1/187\&188}$. I don't want anybody telling me what do do$^{2/437}$. (T)hey're not me mam to make me do$^{2/44}$.'

Editing may also be necessary to clarify the sense and improve readability. Take the following passage from one of our interviews as an example:

'We go every Tuesday . . . his drops. I stopped going though me with him. I have to go everytime with him, every Tuesday. You know like in they go to anybody else's house, health visitors? But she doesn't come here, only once or twice didn't she?'

The edited version might read as follows:

'The health visitor doesn't come here. She only called once or twice. We go every Tuesday to the clinic for Tony's drops. Well, Ted stopped going with me and now I just go with Tony every Tuesday.'

Both these examples illustrate a generic problem in narrative research with inarticulate subjects. Although true to the informant's own words the edited passages convey a false impression of her lucidity. There exists a tension between the intelligibility of the text and the integrity of the subject. In the case of people with learning difficulties this may have repercussions for the credibility of their stories to the reader. One response to our research, for example, has been that the parents couldn't have learning difficulties because they spoke too fluently.

These problems feed into another challenge facing the researcher as editor. How much leeway does he or she have in supplying the words to tell a coherent story? Can researchers loan their subjects the vocabulary they lack to express their thoughts and feelings? How far is an editor allowed to translate people's behaviour into words? These questions assume a crucial significance in the case of subjects who communicate a lot of their meaning in non-verbal ways that cannot otherwise be captured as text. If an informant spits out 'social workers!' and thumps the table, is it acceptable to transcribe this as 'Social workers make me very angry'? If a mother is unable to speak for crying about the memory of having her baby taken away at birth, is it legitimate to write this as, 'I can't speak about it. I can only weep. It still hurts too much.'? And if these two examples do not breach the researcher's obligation of being honest to the data, at exactly what point does the practice of attributing unspoken words to informants become unjustifiable? This issue has reverberations of the controversy sparked by Woodward and Bernstein's use of anonymous sources and unsourced material in their Watergate investigations which some commentators have seen as leading to a Faustian bargain with fiction that paved the way for later journalistic excesses with the truth (as exampled by Woodward's own protegé who won the Pulitzer prize for a feature it later emerged had been made up). The scholastic tradition of sticking closely to the sources puts limits on imagining the world of people with learning difficulties. Editing their stories invites researchers to experiment with ways of representing findings that best capture the experience they wish to convey (Sandelowski 1994).

Interpretation

Editing also involves a process of interpretation. Plummer (1983) draws a contrast between the researcher's and the subject's frame of reference and points out that a key issue in compiling life stories is the weight given to these respective viewpoints. The emphasis shifts from one to the other according to the extent to which the researcher imposes his or her analysis on the subject's raw account. Some researchers object to the analysis of narratives on aesthetic grounds (expounding the message may ruin the story), on political grounds (refusing to acquiese in the power of the audience to whom they are explained) and on the grounds of authenticity (unelaborated stories are more true to people's experiences). Others argue that narratives devoid of analysis do not pass the test of scholarship because they cannot be disputed, and that analysis is needed to move a story beyond the concrete in order to reveal its meaning to people other than the teller (Farber & Sherry 1993).

There are very few unadorned accounts of the lives of people with learning difficulties. The hand of a rapporteur or intermediary is invariably present in their published stories although the steer it exerts varies. The role of the intermediary may be more or less intrusive, ranging on a continuum from *amanuensis* (whose contribution does not alter the text), through *interpreter* (who adds their own construction to the story as told), to *biographer* (who writes about the lives of others in the third person). From this point of view, the problem of interpretation in narrative research goes beyond the role of analysis to embrace the issue of representation. As Bowker (1993) points out, '(e)stablishing "acceptable" versions of lives is as much a political struggle for unknowns as it is for the famous', and people with learning difficulties are ill-placed to challenge the misrepresentation of their experience in the literature. Partly for this reason some scholars have argued for an 'ethics of representation' that would require narrative researchers to make clear who is speaking in their stories.

Ownership

Narrative research with people who have learning difficulties is almost always a collaborative venture. The stories that emerge are usually the product of (at least) two authors: a narrator and a researcher. They are properly seen as 'the creation of two minds working together' (Whittemore *et al.* 1986). This raises the issue of ownership. It may not be possible to completely disentangle the personal threads woven into the stories. Where a researcher helps to elicit the narrative, edits the material, interprets its meaning and converts it into text, the final contribution of the two authors may not be clear. There is a danger of researchers misappropriating (by oversight or design) the lives of the people whose stories are being told.

The issue of ownership is closely related to the problem of implicit conceptualisation or arbitrariness in idiographic research (Allport 1947). Stories can be made to serve many purposes.

Researchers are at risk of imposing their own preconceptions on the raw data: of finding what they are looking for or casting it into a ready-made mould. One example of this kind of pressure is the way the researcher as a 'publisher' of life stories may be thrust into the role of advocate for people or groups otherwise denied a voice (Faraday & Plummer 1979; Bertaux & Kohli 1984). In this case, the question of ownership presents itself in terms of the accountability of researchers to their subjects as against their profession.

These considerations add weight to the importance of upholding a distinction between 'the story' and 'the truth'. As Bowker (1993) has said, 'no faithful method of retrieving biographical "truth" exists'. Every life story is only one among many potential versions and each owes something to the particular relationship from which it springs.

Narrative as an art form

Historians are accustomed to chasing shadows. Dogged by the unavoidable remoteness of their subjects, they are left 'painfully aware of their inability to reconstruct a dead world in its completeness' (Schama 1992). In facing up to this habitual quandary, historians are not averse to exercising their sympathy and intuition in order to supply some of the missing pieces. As Erikson (1973) has pointed out, history more than any other social science recognises that 'the imagination of a disciplined professional mind is itself a research tool of no mean power'.

Sociology has been more inclined to deny a muse. Presented with the same sort of uncertainties that plague historical data, sociologists are prompted by the conventions of their trade to retreat to safer ground where their position can better be defended or their argument more easily substantiated. These same pressures are also seen in the widespread efforts by journal editors and their reviewers to 'scientize qualitative research' (Sandelowski 1994) by insisting that it be reported in a style ill-suited to the genre. The upshot of these instincts has been to retard the development of narrative research as a method of sociological enquiry and, more particularly, to close off access to the subjective worlds of people (such as those with learning difficulties) who are not easily reached using textbook methods and formulaic thinking.

My argument is that sociology needs to become more like history in acknowledging the role of the imagination in the creative reconstruction of other worlds. Its practitioners need to recognise that reality may be apprehended through art as well as science. So far as narrative research is concerned, this entails redefining the boundaries of scholarship to include the fictional form.

There is nothing very challenging about this claim. Nisbet (1962:1976), for example, has argued that a good deal of literature and other art of the age may be seen as 'imaginative forms of sociology'. Great novelists are precisely those whose work throws light on their times. In an article in the *Westminster Review* of 1856, George Eliot wrote that the grand function of art, including novels, is 'the extension of our sympathies': 'it is a mode of amplifying experience and extending our contact with our fellow-men beyond the bounds of our personal lot'. (Pinney 1963). This might almost serve as a maxim for the narrative researcher. George Eliot saw her role as that of an imaginative historian or scientific investigator who seeks to analyse contemporary social and political changes through the human stories she tells (Ashton 1994). It is not a very big leap from this position to the idea that some techniques of the creative writer might in turn be used to breathe life into sociological narratives.

What aspects of the fictional form lend themselves for use by narrative researchers working with inarticulate subjects? Again I shall illustrate the general points by reference to people with learning difficulties.

The use of metaphor

Sociologists are a literal-minded bunch with a mistrust of allegorical styles of discourse. The pursuit of truth, they hold, is not the stuff of legend. Narrative researchers need to rethink this position. After all, a metaphor is a claim about reality (Whale 1984). The virtue of metaphor is that it can seamlessly tie observations together or make an abstract idea visible to the mind's eye. It is tempting to go further and argue that the metaphor serves the narrative equivalent of generalisation by embodying the universal in the particular.

When Rosie Spencer's community nurse took maternity leave she promised to bring the new baby for Rosie to see (cf. Booth & Booth 1994: Chapter 7). When the baby was born, Rosie sent a card and a present. Over twelve months later, Rosie still had not seen him despite her insistent promptings and the community nurse's repeated promises. The saga of Nurse Sharpe's baby came up at some point in almost every conversation throughout this period. Although a seemingly trivial matter in its own right, the story may be read as a metaphor for the devalued status accorded to people with learning difficulties in their dealings with professionals.

Or take Evelyn. She has the habit of seeking reaffirmation by frequently asking, 'Been good?'. It is a mistake to see this trait as a simple craving for praise or approval. Its origins lie in her experience of always having to please the people who run her life or suffer the consequences. 'Been good?' is a metaphor for a lifetime of repression.

Narrative provides researchers with the opportunity to use the elegance and power of metaphor. Although the metaphor needs to be handled with special care, and holds dangers for the unwary, it also presents particular strengths, especially for 'excluded voice' writers who seek to convey ideas in authentic, personal terms rather than through academic prose.

Characterisation

Narrative researchers invariably find themselves trapped between the press of their material and the space for writing it up. The word limit in our contract for *Parenting Under Pressure* meant that we were able to feature in-depth accounts of only four of the seven families who went forward into the second stage of the study (Booth & Booth 1994). Even then they were heavily edited. The first draft of Rosie Spencer's story was almost three times the length of the published version. In abridging the material we were fearful of rendering down Rosie's personality. This is the point at which characterisation shows as a crucial skill.

Characterisation is important in narrative research for at least three reasons. It conveys the storied quality of people's lives and makes it easier for readers to make the imaginative leap into a world beyond their experience. It counteracts the tendency for people to be known only by their labels. Within two pages of Lennie and George's appearance in *Of Mice and Men*, John Steinbeck portrays Lennie's limitations without once pinning a label on him. Narrative researchers too need to learn to write about people as characters rather than types. Characterisation is also a way of coping with the problem of confidentiality in narrative research. Preserving the anonymity of those whose stories are being told becomes more difficult as stories become more detailed. Characterisation may be used to lay false trails that help to mask the subject's identity without distorting their lives.

Composite stories

Composites are characters or stories constructed of parts drawn from more than one original. They may be seen as analytical constructs (or fictions) designed to lend some sort of order to a messy world or to illuminate its darkened corners. As such they bear comparison to Becker's (1940) notion of 'constructed types' that combine selected variables in order to focus attention on the common elements in diverse situations or in people's lives and experience.

Composites may be offered for a variety of reasons. They are a means of coping with the press of material, the constraints of space and the dictates of confidentiality that dog the narrative researcher. They permit the aggregation of partial material from multiple sources, in the same way as a bike might be put together from parts found on a tip. In the case of inarticulate subjects, they may be used to fill out individual narratives to give a fuller picture than any single informant can portray or to piece together a rounded account from snatches of lives.

Life stories are not usually offered for the facts they contain but as sources of understanding. They take particular happenings as their point of reference but, as Bruner (1991) has pointed out, such details are 'their vehicle rather than their destination'. The particularities are important only in so far as they contribute to the general significance of the story. Composites are ways of constructing stories in order to emphasise this emblematic status.

Composites are simultaneously totally true and entirely fictional. They take real-life material and present it in make-believe form. Crafting them involves the exercise of what George Eliot (1963) called a 'veracious imagination' that fills out the evidence by 'careful analogical creation'. As with other constructs, composite stories are not offered as accurate descriptions of empirical reality but for their interpretive or heuristic value. Craig Raine, talking about his book *History: The Home Movie*, says, 'I don't want people to worry about whether it's true or whether it's fiction. I just want them to kind of live in this world – enter it, exist in it, enjoy it.' (Davies 1994). The same might be said of composite stories. The test is not whether they are faithful to the facts (falsifiability) but whether they are true to the subject (verisimilitude). As Sandelowski (1994) has written:

'When you talk with me about my research, do not ask me what I found; I found nothing. Ask me what I invented, what I made up from and out of my data. But know that in asking you to ask me this, I am not confessing to telling any lies about the people or events in my studies/stories. I have told the truth. The proof is in the things I have made – how they look to your mind's eye, whether they satisfy your sense of style and craftsmanship, whether you believe them, and whether they appeal to your heart.'

Dramaturgy

Life stories are productions that call on the dramatic arts of plot, scene, event and action for their successful realisation. Editing lives into text means having regard for the flow, pace, form and structure of the story. Two examples from *Parenting Under*

Pressure illustrate how these considerations bear on the writing of stories.

In Rosie Spencer's case there was insufficient continuous speech to present the story entirely in her words. Accordingly, the researcher's own voice was used to report material not available in the form of first-person narrative. Also her strong present-orientation meant that attention had to be given to what was going on in her life during the course of the fieldwork. This focus led, in turn, to a story structure that reflected the chronology of events as they occurred and in which the researcher loomed large. It is unlikely that Rosie would have given the same prominence to this relationship in recounting the same period in her life to a third party. At the same time, it is not the researcher's story. There is no analysis, the style is straight reportage, and the researcher's perspective is suppressed. The published account is properly seen as the story of a research relationship.

By contrast, Sarah Armstrong's story is presented entirely in her own words. She was one of our most articulate informants whose own voice conveys the pain visited on her family and the strains on her marriage more tellingly than could any professional wordsmith. Her story is structured by the sequence of interviews spanning the twelve months during which her children were taken into care. This serialisation documents the gradual decline of the family into trauma through Sarah's emotions as a wife and mother. For dramatic reasons it was decided not to include her husband Geoff's story. Initially, although prepared to talk freely, he had refused to allow any recording or notetaking. Much of what he had to say was written up afterwards and was not available verbatim. We decided that to mix direct and reported speech would detract from the immediacy of the narrative. Also, while Geoff and Sarah shared the same view of what was happening to them under the pressure of events, Geoff puts a different gloss on his own behaviour. We felt that the dramatic focus of the chapter should be on the breakdown of the family rather than Geoff's conduct.

The published versions of these two stories were each shaped by the tools of the dramatist. Narrative researchers need to develop these skills rather than apologise for them. They are a fundamental part of their method, not a departure from the standards of scientific rigour. Dramaturgy is a way of making real lives comprehensible.

Dialogue

The spoken word does not always transfer easily to the printed page. Even someone with a virtuoso command of the medium of talk like Alastair Cooke has to confess, in a published selection of his letters from America, to 'making the most of the privilege of print to straighten out the syntax' of his broadcasts (Cooke 1980). For people who lack mastery of their own language, the extent of polishing and trimming needed to convey in print the sense and meaning of their conversation can be prodigious.

Dialogue is intimately bound up with the process of characterisation. People reveal themselves through what they say. It is also a vehicle for plot; and for keeping the reader informed, interested and entertained. Again Steinbeck shows the way. Lennie's form of speech is true to the man and friendly to the reader. Narrative researchers need to hone the same skills. Constructing narratives is more than a matter of transcribing interviews and erasing the questions. It entails communicating character and content in a form that is true to the subject while commanding the reader's attention. These are properly the skills of the writer. John Banville, the novelist, makes the point in his review of Parker's (1991) *Life After Life*: 'Tony Parker's material is tape-recorded speech, but he is a very cunning writer. By means of arrangement and pattern, rhythm and tone . . . he makes out of these tape-recorded testimonies a kind of art that is all the more affecting because it springs from fact.'

Faithfully reproducing their spoken words as text may do a gross disservice to people with learning difficulties. Accuracy and the truth do not always go hand in hand. Freed from their contextual supports, loose words easily tumble into chaos. The result may be a false impression of illucidity or the loss of whatever original meaning they carried in conversation. For this reason, narrative researchers should not always seek to preserve the exact form of words their subjects use. Their first duty is to preserve the message those words convey. If this entails redrafting the material using different words in the same idiom they should not spurn the task.

Style

Style is the expression of personality in language. Considerations of style arise for the narrative researcher at three points: when editing the transcript, polishing the text, and when adding a commentary or analysis.

There is a temptation in editing transcripts to excise all material not strictly relevant to the development of the story. Limitations of space often oblige heavy use of the red pen. Yet it is often through such asides that people emerge as personalities. The researcher should make a deliberate effort to ensure that people's individual voices are heard in their stories. Similarly, when polishing the text, care must be taken to maintain the narrator's idiom. The spell is easily broken by writing 'my mother' where the speaker always says 'me mam'.

It should also be remembered that researchers reveal themselves in their writing. People who continue to use terms like 'mental handicap', 'mental deficiency' or 'retardate' against the wishes of those to whom the label is applied are signalling their identification with their professional peers and not with the interests and aspirations of people with learning difficulties. Reading the research literature on parents and parenting it is striking how often authors refer to 'offspring' rather than children, to 'males' and 'females' instead of men and women, to 'mate selection' instead of dating or courting, and to 'mating' or 'coupling' instead of sex. Style shows how people with learning difficulties are still thought of as less than human.

Entertainment and readability

J. H. Plumb, the historian, used to make no secret of the fact that he liked history that could be read as literature. Narrative scholars should aim for no less. As Candia McWilliam (1993) has said, 'All personal accounts of common experience are absorbing.' If narratives fail this test, they have probably failed their subjects. Readability is the key to ensuring that listeners attend the stories. It also has the power to draw readers into a story at an emotional as well as an intellectual level. In the end, narrative researchers, like novelists, who cannot take the reader with them are wasting their time.

Conclusions

Textbook methods of social research discriminate against people with learning difficulties. Methods that rely on reading or writing or abstract reasoning or verbal fluency may effectively exclude them from the role of respondent or informant in ways that mirror their exclusion from the wider society. Wittingly or unwittingly the use of these methods also helps to reinforce the medical model of learning difficulties as individual deficits. Too often the research problem of engaging with people who have learning difficulties is seen in terms of the limitations of the subjects rather than the limitations of conventional research methods. In this way, the research enterprise itself perpetuates a view of disability as individual pathology.

The principal medium of communication for the narrative researcher is words. People who lack mastery of this medium will not have their stories heard unless new ways can be found of giving them a voice. Straight transcriptions of interview material may feed perceptions of personal inadequacy. The argument put forward in this chapter for the development of fictional forms of enquiry is intended as a practical response to the challenge of involving people with learning difficulties as participants in narrative research. At the same time, the fictional form is also commended on political grounds as a way of challenging the medical model of disability that is sustained by methods of research which impose barriers on the participation of people with learning difficulties.

The use of techniques in narrative research more usually associated with the fictional form highlights the need for different criteria of methodological adequacy more suited to this mode of enquiry. Standard tests such as reliability, validity and replicability are neither appropriate nor adequate when lives are not consistent, biographical truth is a will-o'-the-wisp and stories inevitably reflect something of the teller. Narratives may be better judged by aesthetic standards (Abrams 1991), by their emotive force or their capacity to engage the reader emotionally in the story being told, by their verisimilitude rather than their verifiability (Bruner 1991) and by criteria of authenticity or integrity concerned with how far stories are true to the lives of those they portray. The elaboration of these criteria is a task that remains to be pursued within the sociology of disability.

References

Abrams, K. (1991) 'Hearing the call of stories' *California Law Review*, 79, pp. 971–1052.

Allport, G. (1947) *The Use of Personal Documents in Psychological Science* (Bull. 49). New York: Social Science Research Council.

Ashe, M. (1989) 'Zig-zag stitching and the seamless web: thoughts on "reproduction" and the law' *Nova Law Review*, 13, pp. 355–83.

Ashton, R. (1994) 'Introduction' to the Penguin edition of George Eliot's *Middlemarch*.

Baron, J. (1991) 'The many promises of storytelling in law'. *Rutgers Law Journal*, 23, pp. 79–105.

Becker, H. (1940) 'Constructive typology in the social sciences' in H. Barnes, H. Becker and F. Becker (eds.), *Contemporary Social Theory*. New York: Appleton-Century.

Bertaux, D. and Kohli, M. (1984) 'The life story approach: a continental view' *American Review of Sociology*, 10, pp. 215–37.

Bertaux, D. (1981) 'Introduction' in D. Bertaux (ed.), *Biography and Society*. London: Sage Publications.

Bertaux-Wiame, I. (1981) 'The life-history approach to the study of internal migration' in D. Bertaux (ed.), *Biography and Society*. London: Sage Publications.

Birren, J. and Deutchman, D. (1991) *Guiding Autobiography Groups for Older Adults*. London: The John Hopkins University Press.

Bogdan, R. (1974) *Being Different: The Autobiography of Jane Fry*. London: Wiley.

Booth, T. and Booth, W. (1994) *Parenting Under Pressure: Mothers and Fathers with Learning Difficulties.* Buckingham: Open University Press.

Booth, T., Simons, K. and Booth, W. (1990) *Outward Bound: Relocation and Community Care for People with Learning Difficulties.* Buckingham: Open University Press.

Booth, W. and Fielden, S. (1992) Second opinions: students' views of Swallow Street Centre. Unpublished report, Department of Sociological Studies, University of Sheffield.

Bowker, G. (1993) 'The age of biography is upon us' *The Times Higher Education Supplement*, January 8, p. 19.

Brandon, D. and Ridley, J. (1983) *Beginning to Listen – A Study of the Views of Residents Living in a Hostel for Mentally Handicapped People.* London: MIND.

Cattermole, M., Jahoda, A. and Markova, J. (1987) *Leaving Home: The Experience of People with a Mental Handicap*, Department of Psychology, University of Stirling.

Connerton, P. (1989) *How Societies Remember.* Cambridge: Cambridge University Press.

Cooke, A. (1980) *The Americans: Letters from America 1969–1979.* Harmondsworth: Penguin.

Davies, J. (1994) (An interview with Craig Raine). *The Times Higher*, 9 September, p. 16.

Denzin, N. (1989) *Interpretive Biography.* London: Sage.

Edgerton, R., Bollinger, M. and Herr, B. (1984) 'The cloak of competence: after two decades', *American Journal of Mental Deficiency*, 88(4), pp. 345–51.

Eliot, G. (1963) 'Leaves from a note-book: historical imagination', in T. Pinney (Ed.) *Essays of George Eliot.* London: Routledge and Kegan Paul.

Erikson, K. (1973) 'Sociology and the historical perspective' in M. Drake (ed.) *Applied Historical Studies.* London: Methuen in association with Open University Press.

Faraday, A. and Plummer, K. (1979) 'Doing life histories' *Sociological Review*, 27, pp. 773–98.

Farber, D. and Sherry, S. (1993) 'Telling stories out of school: an essay on legal narratives' *Stanford Law Review*, 45, pp. 807–55.

Ferrarotti, F. (1981) 'On the autonomy of the biographical method' in D. Bertaux (ed.), *Biography and Society.* London: Sage Publications.

Flynn, M. (1989) *Independent Living for Adults with Mental Handicap.* London: Cassell.

Lewis, O. (1961) *Children of Sanchez: Autobiography of a Mexican Family.* New York: Random House.

Lowe, K., de Paiva, S. and Humphreys, S. (1986) *Long Term Evaluations of Services for People with a Mental Handicap in Cardiff: Clients' Views*, Mental Handicap in Wales – Applied Research Unit.

McWilliam, C. (1993) (Review of *Women as Revolutionary Agents of Change*). *Independent on Sunday*, 21 February, p. 28.

Malin, N. (1983) *Group Homes for Mentally Handicapped People.* London: HMSO.

Mount, B. and Zwernik, K. (1988) *It's Never Too Early, It's Never Too Late: A Booklet about Personal Futures Planning*, Publication No. 421-88-109, Metropolitan Council, Minnesota, USA.

Nisbet, R. (1962) 'Sociology as an art form' *Pacific Sociological Review*, 5, pp. 67–74.

Nisbet, R. (1976) *Sociology as an Art Form*. London: Heinemann.

Parker, T. (1991) *Life After Life*. London: Pan Books.

Passfield, D. (1983) 'What do you think of it so far? A survey of 20 Priory Court residents' *Mental Handicap*, 11(3), pp. 97–9.

Pinney, T. (ed.) (1963) *Essays of George Eliot*. London: Routledge and Kegan Paul.

Plummer, K. (1983) *Documents of Life*. London: Allen and Unwin.

Potts, M. and Fido, R. (1990) *They Take My Character*. Plymouth: Northcote House.

Richards, S. (1984) *Community Care of the Mentally Handicapped: Consumer Perspectives*, University of Birmingham.

Sandelowski, M. (1994) 'The proof is in the pottery: towards a poetic for qualitative inquiry' in J. Morse (ed.), *Critical Issues in Qualitative Research Methods*. London: Sage.

Schama, S. (1991) *Dead Certainties (Unwarranted Speculations)*. London: Granta Books.

Spradley, J. (1979) *The Ethnographic Interview*. London: Holt, Rinehart and Winston.

Sugg, B. (1987) 'Community care: the consumer's point of view', *Community Care*, 645, 22 January, p. 6.

Warshaw, R. (1989) *I Never Called It Rape*. New York: Harper and Row.

Welsh Office (1991) *The Review of the All Wales Strategy: A View from the Users*. Cardiff: Social Services Inspectorate.

Whale, J. (1984) *Put It In Writing*. London: Dent.

Whittemore, R., Langness, L. and Koegel, P. (1986) 'The life history approach to mental retardation' in L. Langness and H. Levine (eds.), *Culture and Retardation*, Kluwer, D. Reidel Publishing Company.

Williams, P. (1991) *The Alchemy of Race and Rights: The Diary of a Law Professor*. Cambridge: Harvard University Press.

INDEX